The Ultimate Gluten-Free Cookie Book

Also by Roben Ryberg:

You Won't Believe It's Gluten-Free!

The Gluten-Free Kitchen

Recipes by Roben Ryberg:

Eating for Autism

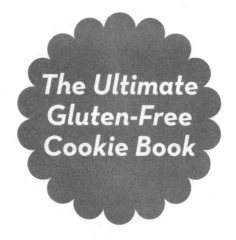

The Ultimate Gluten-Free Cookie Book

125 FAVORITE RECIPES

Roben Ryberg

Da Capo
LIFE
LONG

A Member of the Perseus Books Group

Designed by Pauline Brown
Set in 12 point Goudy Old Style by the Perseus Books Group

Library of Congress Cataloging-in-Publication Data

Ryberg, Roben.
    The ultimate gluten-free cookie book : 125 favorite recipes / Roben Ryberg.—1st Da Capo Press ed.
        p. cm.
    Includes index.
    ISBN 978-0-7382-1376-7 (pbk. : alk. paper) 1. Gluten-free diet—Recipes. I. Title.
RM237.86.R932 2010
641.5'638—dc22
                                2010029918

First Da Capo Press edition 2010
ISBN: 978-0-7382-1376-7

Published by Da Capo Press
A Member of the Perseus Books Group
www.dacapopress.com

Da Capo Press books are available at special discounts for bulk purchases in the U.S. by corporations, institutions, and other organi-zations. For more information, please contact the Special Markets Department at the Perseus Books Group, 2300 Chestnut Street, Suite 200, Philadelphia, PA, 19103, or call (800) 810-4145, ext. 5000, or e-mail special .markets@perseusbooks.com.

10 9 8 7 6 5 4 3 2 1

To happy days,
counting blessings
old and new . . .

Contents

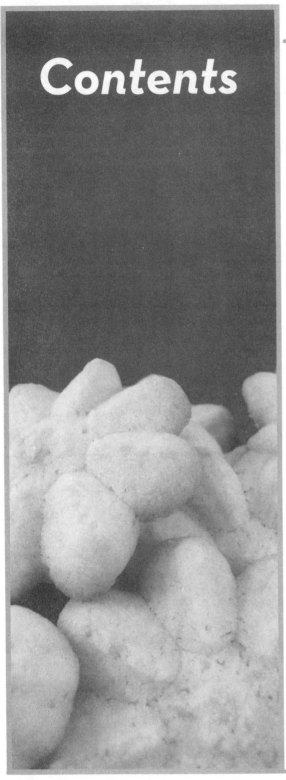

Butter Cookies, page 67

4 **Bar Cookies, 41**

5 **Rolled and Piped Cookies, 65**

6 **Great Fakes Cookies, 93**

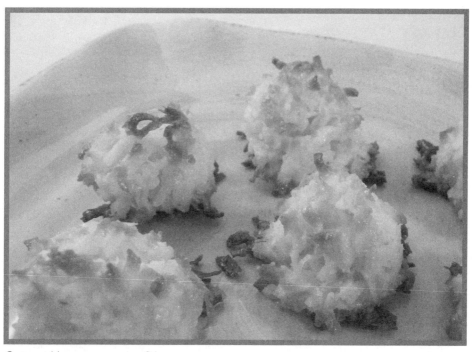

Coconut Macaroons, page 26

Acknowledgments

To those that guide my research:

Thank you for your feedback on gluten-free foods; for wanting healthier, whole-grain flours; for demanding good taste; and for wanting foods that don't stale in just one day. Thank you for pushing me to do better simply.

To those that test:

Thank you to the Boonsboro High School cross-country team for eating batch after batch of cookies; to friends who took cookies to bake sales to raise awareness of gluten sensitivity; to Crawford's diner for testing and sharing my cookies with customers; to other friends and family for fearlessly testing again and again.

To those that give:

Thank you to Sara Boswell for sharing her expertise in food science; to Stacie Nitza, my fellow foodie; to Cassandra Gee for baking, editing, and playing cheerleader; to the gluten-free community, both online and in various states, for supporting my work; to the Girl Scouts of Central Maryland, Inc., for providing samples of their cookies so that I could test my "great fakes" side-by-side with their outstanding cookies.

Foreword

By Dr. Stephen Wangen

Roben and I first met at a national conference on gluten intolerance sponsored by GIG, the Gluten Intolerance Group of North America (www.gluten.net). Like everyone there, we shared a keen interest in everything gluten-free.

Roben has a passion for making gluten-free bread and baked goods. However, she isn't satisfied with "good" alternatives. She demands that they are as close to the real thing as possible. In a recent conversation where she was describing the painstaking process that she went through to develop one particular cookie, I was impressed with her persistence and her patience. She spent hours coming up with just the right mix of ingredients and techniques to perfectly replicate a traditional cookie. And that was just one of the more than one hundred cookies in this book!

We also share an interest in the significant health benefits of being gluten-free. My passion is in helping people to discover their gluten intolerance. Too many people remain undiagnosed. And many people think that gluten intolerance and celiac disease are essentially the same thing. But celiac disease only represents a fraction of those who are gluten intolerant.

Celiac disease is caused by an inability to digest gluten, a protein found in wheat, rye, (cross-contaminated) oats, and barley. This condition affects about 1 percent of the population, or around 3 million people in the United States. These people develop damage in the small intestine called villous atrophy. However, there are millions more who are suffering from gluten intolerance who do not get this type of damage in the small intestine because it only represents one possible result of a gluten intolerance. These people often get overlooked or misdiagnosed, as do many people who have celiac disease. As a medical community doctors are still only in the early stages of properly recognizing this problem.

It is worth noting that nonceliac gluten intolerance is not necessarily any less severe than that of celiac disease. And in many people it is more severe. In either case, avoiding gluten helps to resolve an incredibly large number of health problems. There are well over two hundred different conditions known to be associated with gluten intolerance, and the list grows weekly as more research is done. Many common complaints such as fatigue, headaches, arthritis, anemia, heartburn, diarrhea, constipation, gas, bloating, abdominal pain, eczema, osteoporosis, and even weight gain can be caused by a gluten intolerance. A more complete list can be found in my new book, *Healthier Without Wheat: A New Understanding of Wheat Allergies, Celiac Disease, and Non-Celiac Gluten Intolerance*.

Of course, going gluten-free is easier said than done. This is where the ideal of living healthier without gluten meets the practicality of trying to do just that. It's a steep learning curve, and there are bound to be frustrations. There are also the emotional attachments to food that we develop over a lifetime. And that is never truer than it is for baking cookies, which is almost a national pastime.

For these reasons, we are incredibly fortunate to have Roben's book. Roben has dramatically shortened the learning curve for the rest of us, and given us hope that we can maintain some old traditions as long as we're willing to learn to do them a little differently. And she has done this for just about any cookie that one can imagine, or at least that I can imagine.

What's more, Roben has also incorporated the recent research by the Cereal Quality Lab at Texas A&M to bring us a healthier cookie. That may sound like a bit of an oxymoron, but every effort helps. Gluten-free foods are nutritionally often a shell of their wheat-based counterparts. Using brown rice flour and sorghum flour is a major improvement, and it doesn't detract from the taste of the cookie. These are still the real thing, not some health food substitute for a cookie.

I hope that you enjoy learning to bake these cookies, and I am thrilled that you'll be able to be gluten-free in the process. On behalf of all of us, thank you, Roben.

Dr. Stephen Wangen
www.HealthierWithoutWheat.com

The Science of Gluten-Free Cookies

By Texas A&M University, Cereal Quality Lab, College Station, TX

Carbon, hydrogen, oxygen—no, we are not in chemistry class. We are discussing the elemental ingredients in your cookies. A certain fuzzy blue monster once sang, "C is for Cookie and that's good enough for me," but when it comes to baking easy gluten-free and allergy-free cookies, one has to take a closer look at the science behind the combination of ingredients that we are using.

Your typical wheat-based cookie is made from what bakers call "soft flour." A soft flour means that it has a lower protein (gluten) content than a hard wheat flour that is used to make wheat breads. The gluten protein in the flour helps hold the dough and the final cookie or bread together. That's why your cookie is soft and easy to chew but strong enough to keep from crumbling. Gluten-free baking can often be frustrating, as you no longer have the majority of that protein structure. Gluten-free flours do not have the same type of proteins that hold your other contents together, so ingredients like xanthan gum or guar gum are added to gluten-free dough to help out instead. Fortunately, due to the low gluten content in cookie recipes, cookies are easier to mimic for gluten-free recipes than more complicated products.

Gluten-free flours are made from a wide variety of grains, pseudo-grains, seeds, nuts, tubers, and pretty much anything else you can think of that can be ground into a semi-powder form to be called a "flour." Some gluten-free flours are processed into what is sold as a starch, just a portion of the parent flour. These starches (sometimes referred to as flours by producers) from potato, tapioca, and corn are often criticized for being "unhealthy," so this poses the questions: What is starch? And why does it make my gluten-free baked goods tasty?

Starch is the primary constituent of all cookies, gluten-free or not. It is a naturally occurring carbohydrate found in fruits, vegetables, grains, and tubers that are made up of thousands upon thousands of glucose molecules linked together. The easiest way to visualize starch in its natural form is to grab a sheet of paper and draw a circle on it; this is your starch granule that is made up of the thousands of little glucose molecules. Any flour, when you look at it under a microscope, contains lots of these starch granules that make up the "bulk" of what you can see and feel of the flour.

Starch can take many different sizes, shapes, and forms depending on the source you are using, but they don't act the same. For instance, the starch in tapioca is not the same as the starch in rice. Some starch granules can be shaped like pentagons, some in nice round circles or ovals, and the sizes vary as well. In baking, when liquid is added to the batter or dough and then heated, the starch molecules soak up the water molecules, causing the chemical bonds within the starch to change. When the water-soaked starch reaches a certain temperature it melts (gelatinizes), which means that you can no longer see the original shape of the starch granule and it helps hold the crumb of the cookie or bread you are baking together, like glue. Starch, whether used in pure form or as a component of all flours, is a critical part of gluten-free baking as it makes up for the majority of the structure of your cookie or bread, since the traditional wheat proteins are missing.

The cookie recipes that Roben created for this book mainly use brown rice flour or sorghum flour. These are two easy to find, high fiber, nutritious, and economical flours. Her recipes will not fill your pantry with expensive flours often utilized in various gluten-free blends. We hope that you enjoy the recipes from this book as much as we do—and remember, you don't need seven different kinds of flour to make a good cookie!

Sara Boswell, Research Assistant
Cassandra McDonough, M.S., Research Scientist
Dr. Lloyd Rooney, Regents Professor and Faculty Fellow
Texas A&M University, Cereal Quality Lab, College Station, TX

Introduction

As I write these words, I think about you standing there, trying to figure out which gluten-free cookbook to buy and wondering if these cookies will taste good. You may even be wondering if purchasing ingredients will stress your budget, too. I wish you could be in my kitchen, having the scent of delicious, fresh-baked cookies hit you as you enter my home, and sampling three or four kinds while we chat. But you'll have to settle for my words, my reputation, and my photos. The picture of Girl Scout Thin Mints–Style Cookies on page 6 of the insert, one of my favorite great fakes, is representative that almost anything is deliciously possible in a gluten-free cookie.

Whether seeking a squishy scooter pie, a delicate butter cookie, or a crisp graham cracker, you will find it here. I thought about making a separate chapter for dairy-free cookies, but most of the cookies in this book are dairy-free. Dairy just doesn't always enhance a gluten-free cookie recipe. I have, however, made a separate chapter for egg-free cookies. In that chapter I opt to avoid egg substitutes and, as in the rest of this book, use ordinary ingredients to tempt your taste buds.

These amazing cookies are not only easy to make, they're as close as you can get to the real deal. I've been working in the gluten-free industry since the early 1990s, but I myself do not live with major dietary restrictions (although I limit dairy). I am a food science junkie and a person that simply loves food. I will test, test, and retest a gluten-free recipe until the nuances are achieved, often by eating the original alongside my version. I don't have to remember or wonder what something tastes like (although some foods are vivid in everyone's memory!). I simply taste the original cookie, dissect it, and do my best to duplicate the experience for you.

In the last thirty years, gluten-free baking has come a long way. (See Chapter 1 for a discussion of the evolution of gluten-free baking and how we ended up with complicated food.) Fortunately, by embracing food science and daring to think simpler, we now can have delicious, healthier treats, made with just *one* bag of flour, a little xanthan gum, and everyday ingredients already in your kitchen.

Most of the cookies in this book are made with either brown rice flour or sorghum. Really—that's it! No complicated flour blends required. All I can say, is how cool is that? Brown rice flour is a healthy, affordable, whole-grain flour that provides a wonderful, neutral base on which to build cookie flavor! Sorghum flour, nearly whole-grain, has a lower glycemic index, good nutrition, and an understated fuller grain flavor that doesn't spar with other flavors. And both of these flours can produce incredible textures!

Setting aside food science, it just feels great knowing that you will have tasty cookies! But hopefully, this book gives you something more . . . fabulous cookies to take to a party, a marathon holiday baking session with loved ones, s'mores at a backyard barbecue, renewed fame for cookie-baking talents, or the most sought-after cookies on the tray. It is my goal that this book brings you the simple joy of cookies. And when you taste your first scrumptious cookie from this book, know that I'm smiling with you. Cookie, cookies, cookies. Life can be sweet.

1

Successful Gluten-Free Baking

I first began experimenting with gluten-free foods nearly two decades ago, when a friend of mine who was diagnosed with gluten intolerance innocently asked me if I could help make her something tasty to eat. At that time many gluten-free recipes were made with just rice flour. They were often gritty, dried out quickly, and didn't taste very good. Availability was sparse and the industry was just taking notice of the need for gluten-free foods.

Over the last fifteen years or so, thanks to advances in food science, gluten-free baking has evolved to produce really delicious desserts. These results were made possible by using blends of two, three, four . . . or even seven different alternative flours. Sometimes gelatin, ascorbic acid, and other ingredients were added to provide better results. And, to their credit, many recipes and gluten-free cookbooks use blends that create admirable products.

But using many different flours in a blend can quickly get complicated for you, the baker. After all, who wants to buy three different kinds of expensive flour to make one recipe, then several other flours to make another? Did the pendulum have to swing so far in such a difficult direction? Why choose complicated? So, I began to work toward improving single-flour gluten-free baking. And as it turns out, it can be done very successfully!

About Flour Blends

Historically we've found that those early, simple gluten-free baking recipes provided less than ideal results. Complicated recipes that called for multiple grains and starches were more reliable. But why? Are complex blends really necessary?

First we must understand why blends work. It has everything to do with flour textures and baking properties. To oversimplify, if you think of a cup of traditional white (wheat) flour, you could say it is a perfect 5 on a scale of 1 to 10! Utilizing traditional white flour makes cakes and cookies that turn out just as we expect.

Traditional white flour is not too light, not too heavy. Accordingly, if you're baking cookies, this perfect 5 would beat out a 10—a light flour that rises greatly and which would be at the highest end of our scale—anytime. Likewise, a 2 or a 3 "heavy" flour (at the bottom of our scale) wouldn't be good, either. And, as early history has proven, a heavy flour, such as rice, substituted in a recipe cup for cup, would typically result in baked goods with a texture like a hockey puck or cardboard. It is funny only in hindsight!

Although using blends is generally not my philosophy, let's see how one is made. Remember that 5 is the known perfect on our scale. If you were to take one or more light alternative flours (such as tapioca starch, potato starch, or cornstarch) and combine them with several heavier flours (such as cornmeal, brown rice flour, or millet), you would end up with an averaged value pretty close to perfect. To take a very broad view, light flours = 10, heavy flours = 1. Add 10 plus 1 and then divide by 2, and you have just about achieved the perfect 5.

But it doesn't stop there. While we're building a better mousetrap, let's worry about empty flours (starches with limited dietary benefit—but easy on a tender gut), fiber levels (whole grains, flax, and others), protein levels (think soy and bean flours), and more attributes of other pseudograins! If you combine all these levels of flours, some light, some medium, some heavy, you can still stay near that perfect 5 and enhance nutrition at the same time!

Wow, all of that in a flour blend! If flour represented our entire dietary intake (and if it were the only ingredient in a recipe), that would be ideal. We do, however, eat other nutritious foods. Have we ever expected so much from traditional breads, cakes, and cookies?

Should you choose to mix blends to use for baking, you will soon find your cupboards full of alternative flours. It may be difficult to evaluate which of them your body tolerates. It may be also difficult to know the true flavor of some of these flours, because they are part of a blend. Sometimes we can look at the source of the flour and get a feel for how it will taste. Bean flour does, actually, taste like beans. Coconut flour tastes like coconut with every bit of sweet juice removed (like tropical dirt, in my opinion). And some others taste worse (soy tastes like grass, montina like dried corn husks—actually good in a small quantity; quinoa even grassier; teff is earthy and grassy; etc.). I'm just sharing my honest opinions before you spend a lot of money on a flour you may not enjoy. Although one can make a cookie out of almost anything, that doesn't mean you want to eat it.

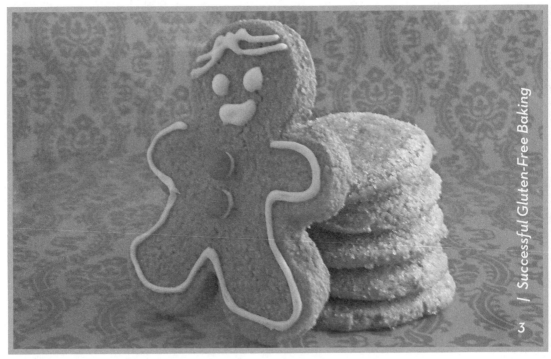

Gingerbread Men and Gingersnaps, page 81

And, let us not forget the irony of giving a person with a sensitive immune system a flour blend that contains several flours that are among the top eight allergens in the United States,* for instance, tree nuts (e.g., almonds) or soybeans. And dare we further consider people with multiple food allergies, such as to dairy, eggs (both also among those top eight allergens), and corn? Does this make sense?

Alternatively, we have a simple solution. Use just one flour and use it in ratios that make sense. Don't just take a regular recipe and substitute the flour cup for cup. Instead, I've developed recipes that embrace and maximize that flour's unique characteristics and baking properties. Let's stop treating an apple like a banana!

Gluten-Free Baking Simplified

I have listened closely to food concerns from the gluten-free community. In my first book, *The Gluten-Free Kitchen*, great taste was the primary goal (and of course, remains so today). I utilized cornstarch and potato starch to make foods that closely resembled their traditional counterparts. It was my goal to make the reader eat safely, not feel deprived, and finally, eat other nutritious foods to round out a healthy diet.

The recipes in my second book, *You Won't Believe It's Gluten-Free!* utilized one flour at a time to create almost any food desired. Cornstarch alone, potato starch alone, rice flour alone, and oat flour alone. It provided the reader with an opportunity to figure out what suited their taste buds and their gut. It also provided a huge array of everyday foods from appetizers to desserts.

My third major work, as contributing food writer for *Eating for Autism*, pushed my gluten-free food making knowledge to the limits. Nutritious, dairy-free, soy-free, corn-free, refined sugar-free, etc. It forced me to rethink our gluten-free base flours once again. Ultimately a combination of brown

---

* www.fda.gov/Food/FoodSafety/FoodAllergens

rice flour and sorghum became a new proving ground for the special dietary guidelines suggested in this work. It was groundbreaking and delicious.

And, that brings us to today. I am delighted to tell you that the recipes in *The Ultimate Gluten-Free Cookie Book* primarily use brown rice flour or sorghum flour. Most often they are used just one at a time. If you had asked me as little as two years ago if any heavy flour could be used to make a cookie that is light and fluffy, such as whoopie pies, I would have said, "Impossible." Today I know it is a reality!

Exploiting the unique characteristics of each of these flours makes "light and fluffy" possible. Also, "tender and crisp." The same goes for "soft and tender." These cookie qualities are all possible using nearly *any* flour (or any blend, for that matter). The final chapter in this book uses other flours solo to make that point. Hopefully, those recipes will also enable you to use up that cupboard full of alternatives fondly called a tower of flours!

For good taste, great textures, good nutrition, and reasonable affordability, I am embracing the wonderful and hard-to-believe attributes of brown rice flour and sorghum flour.

The Cost of Flours

From the CSA/USA Web site (www.csaceliacs.org), I gathered five well-known blend formulas. From the Bob's Red Mill Web site (www.bobs redmill.com), I gathered pricing information for types of flours sometimes used in gluten-free baking. The point in gathering this information is to show how purchase of multiple flours can quickly become quite an expense (not to mention utilize cabinet space!)*

---

* The cost of xanthan gum is not included in the analysis of these blends. That would add an additional cost of $11.96 per 8-ounce package. A package of xanthan gum lasts a very long time! Nor do any of these blends contain some of the more recently embraced alternative flours, which are typically quite costly and would substantially increase the cost.

TABLE 1.1 THE COST OF FLOURS

almond meal	$11.53	1 pound	4 cups	$2.88 per cup
amaranath flour	$7.55	1.5 pounds	5 cups	$1.51 per cup
brown rice flour	$3.03	1.5 pounds	4.25 cups	$.71 per cup
buckwheat	$3.56	1.5 pounds	5 cups	$.71 per cup
coconut flour	$6.92	1 pound	4 cups	$1.73 per cup
cornstarch	$2.29	1.5 pounds	4.8 cups	$.48 per cup
flaxseed meal	$3.06	1 pound	4.25 cups	$.72 per cup
garfava bean	$8.17	1.5 pounds	5 cups	$1.63 per cup
millet flour	$2.72	1.5 pounds	5.25 cups	$.52 per cup
potato flour	$5.66	1.5 pounds	60 tbsp	$.09 per tbsp
potato starch	$3.01	1.5 pounds	3.5 cups	$.86 per cup
quinoa flour	$10.10	1.5 pounds	5.5 cups	$1.84 per cup
sorghum flour	$3.01	1.5 pounds	4.5 cups	$.67 per cup
soy flour	$2.19	1 pound	4 cups	$.55 per cup
tapioca starch/flour	$2.25	1.25 pounds	5 cups	$.45 per cup
teff flour	$6.81	1.5 pounds	5.5 cups	$1.24 per cup
white rice flour	$2.44	1.5 pounds	4.25 cups	$.57 per cup
xanthan gum	$11.96	8 ounces (used in small quantity)		
gluten-free, all-purpose, baking mix	$3.67	1.5 pounds	5 cups	$.73 per cup

GENERAL BAKING MIX #1
Carol Fenster
(makes 2 cups)

1 cup rice flour

½ to ¾ cup potato starch

¼ cup tapioca starch

Initial cost for flours = $7.70; $0.62 per cup

GENERAL BAKING MIX #2
Carol Fenster
(makes 9 cups)

3 cups garfava bean

2 cups potato starch

2 cups cornstarch

1 cup tapioca flour

1 cup sorghum flour

Initial cost for flours = $18.73; $0.91 per cup

ORIGINAL FORMULA
Bette Hagman
(makes 3 cups)

2 cups rice flour

⅔ cup potato starch

⅓ cup tapioca starch

Initial cost for flours = $7.70; $0.66 per cup

FOUR FLOUR BEAN
Bette Hagman
(makes 3 cups)

⅔ cup garfava bean flour

⅓ cup sorghum flour

1 cup cornstarch

1 cup tapioca starch

Initial cost for flours = $15.72; $0.93 per cup

FEATHERLIGHT
Bette Hagman
(makes 3 cups)

1 cup rice flour

1 cup cornstarch

1 cup tapioca starch

1 tablespoon potato flour

Initial cost for flours = $12.64; $0.53 per cup.

Alternatively, a 1.5-pound bag of brown rice flour or sorghum flour costs about $3.00, or roughly $0.70 per cup.

And, finally, factor in the ratios of flours used. Blends are often substituted cup for cup; not so for my single-flour recipes. For example, a traditional chocolate cake may call for 1¾ cups of flour in addition to the cocoa. Two versions of chocolate cakes (in *You Won't Believe It's Gluten-Free!*) use just 3/4 cup of potato starch or 1 cup of rice flour. Food science tells us that our ratios do not need to mirror the rules of traditional baking. Gluten-free flours should have their own rules!

Obviously, we don't need to spend a lot on flours to bake delicious treats! Specifically, we only need one flour (or two if you like), a package of xanthan gum (used in very small quantity, so it lasts for a long time), and an adventurous spirit.

We don't need more blends. We don't need all of our nutritional needs met with unusual-tasting pseudograins. We don't need yet another flour discovery. We need common sense. Let us enjoy the whole-grain goodness of brown rice flour and sorghum flour.* This book lets you set aside venturing into many flour directions (and avoid the, shall we say, interesting taste of many), and make some great cookies!

Making a Great Gluten-Free Cookie

The cookie recipes in this book are, for the most part, quite easy to make. There is science behind the ratios, the choice of ingredients, and the order in which the ingredients are mixed.

To ensure success, first, measure the ingredients carefully. A scale provides more accurate measurements, but is not essential. Combine the sugar and fat and mix well. Scrape down the sides of the bowl.

---

* Often referred to as whole grain by many, sorghum is technically not whole grain, but carries many nutritious properties.

| The Ultimate Gluten-Free Cookie Book

8

Add the flour and mix well. This step is critical, even though your dough just looks like crumbles in the mixing bowl. Essentially, you are coating the individual flour particles with fat, thereby deterring the flour from stealing moistness from the finished cookie. This simple step greatly extends the moistness-life of any gluten-free cookie (or any other baked good for that matter!). This step also helps a cookie to retain its intended character. (For example, a crisp cookie can become soft in a day if this step is not followed!)

Add the remaining ingredients as directed. You don't have to worry too much about overbeating the batter as there is no gluten in our flours. It is the gluten that develops in traditional flour when you overbeat it, which can make a cookie tough. However, excess beating may cause increased viscosity of the xanthan gum, making the finished cookie hold shape a little stronger than desired. But the taste and texture should not change!

For rolled cookies, I strongly recommend a lightly oiled surface and rolling pin. We don't want to add any dryness (flour) to the exterior of our cookies! Gluten-free cookie dough may require a small amount of shaping with moist fingertips to have finished results that mirror their traditional counterparts.

Bake at the recommended temperature. Do not be tempted to speed along baking with a higher temperature. Browning and spread are both affected by temperature!

Finally, it is best to avoid substitutions in a recipe. If you can, try the recipe as written the first time and venture from there. The helpful hints that follow should help you as you become more adventurous in your baking.

Helpful Hints

With each new cookbook I write, unwritten rules of gluten-free food theory become clear. I first disclosed a set of gluten-free food theories and helpful hints while speaking at a celiac conference in Dallas. It was my most popular handout, and requests for copies even followed me home. Following are my latest gluten-free cookie baking theories and helpful hints.

Fats

1. Shortening makes for the crispest cookie. Butter makes for the richest and even a little softer cookie. Oil makes for a crisp and tender cookie. These are subtle differences, but very important depending upon the desired result.

2. Coating a flour with fat first dramatically extends the moisture-life of the baked item.

3. Use margarine with at least 80 percent fat if substituting for butter.

Sweeteners

1. Sweeteners entirely change a cookie. Sugar makes for a dryer cookie. Honey makes for a soft cookie.

2. Sugar can be baked at a higher temperature than honey without burning. If using honey and you want a crisp cookie, you need a low temperature for a much longer time.

3. Honey tastes sweeter than corn syrup.

4. In some cookies, such as the animal crackers, you would think that you'd want sugar to produce that nice crisp texture. Not when you are baking with brown rice flour; using sugar throws you into a sugar cookie taste and texture. You must have honey, which adds the complication of how to get a cookie that's soft, but dry. Yes, I know they are crisp, but the starting dough is soft and the edges need to soften when baking. The honey also makes for tenderness.

Eggs

1. Egg-free cookies benefit from additional moist ingredients such as pumpkin or applesauce.

2. Using honey or corn syrup makes eggs less necessary in a recipe.

Flours

1. Tenderness is achieved with rice flour by using oil as the fat.
2. Rice flour carries the flavor of butter extraordinarily well, so less butter can be used.
3. Peanut butter must be viewed as both a fat and a flour. To oversimplify, consider 50 percent by volume as fat and 50 percent as solids (the latter, as you would a flour).
4. Lighten a recipe by using starch in place of some of the gritty flour. Or use extra egg whites, leavening, etc.

Binding

1. Gluten-free dough wants to bind itself to fillings or toppings. While cookies will still be delicious assembled together, prebaking can help maintain the separateness of components. A gluten-free dough that has corn syrup as the sweetener is not as likely to bind itself to fillings. (See the Rugalach recipe, page 138.)
2. Cornstarch as a thickener is not as effective in the presence of an acid (such as lemon).
3. Xanthan gum does not exhibit strong binding properties when egg yolks are the only "liquid" in a recipe.
4. Xanthan gum exhibits stronger binding properties to a water-based liquid than to oil. (This may be the reason some of you notice a spongier texture in commercially available mixes, when replacing part of the fat with applesauce—acting as a water-based liquid.)
5. Xanthan gum exhibits stronger binding properties to corn syrup than to honey.
6. Use less xanthan gum if switching from dairy- to water-based liquids.
7. Xanthan gum has greater viscosity in the bowl than does guar gum. Guar gum has a greater binding effect in the oven. Guar gum can have a laxative effect.
8. Substitute $1^{1}/_{4}$ teaspoons of guar gum for 1 teaspoon of xanthan gum.

9. Not all xanthan gums are created equal! Surprisingly, some brands have less binding capabilities than others! Even the same brand can have an off batch on occasion.

10. Not all xanthan gum is grown on a corn base. Historically, some xanthan, grown on sugar cane base, has been available. Recently, it has been difficult to locate.

Rising

1. Not all baking powders are created equal! Rumford provides more action in the bowl as compared to Clabber Girl. Clabber Girl provides more action in the oven. You may need to reduce baking powder by 25 percent if not using Rumford.

2. Baking soda is four times stronger than baking powder and needs an acid to activate. Acids include vinegar, yogurt, brown sugar, cocoa powder, and lemon juice.

Miscellaneous

1. Use the same brand of ingredients as does the writer of the recipe, whenever possible, especially when first trying an author's work.

2. Generally speaking, don't worry about overbeating doughs and batters as there is no gluten to develop. Note, however, extensive beating can increase the viscosity of xanthan gum, making for a thicker dough or batter.

3. The use of sugar and/or baking soda in a recipe helps browning.

2

Kitchen and Baking Tips

Even if you are an experienced baker, I hope you will take a few minutes to peruse this chapter! While some things may be obvious, I hope to give you a feel for the methods and equipment used frequently in this book to make great gluten-free cookies.

Cleanliness and Preventing Cross-Contamination

Without safeguards, lovingly prepared food can be dangerous to a person living with gluten-intolerance or celiac disease, as even the smallest traces of gluten must be avoided. To avoid cross-contamination, it is critical that your kitchen be a safe preparation and cooking area. The thought of wayward crumbs or flying flour dust is enough to make someone with celiac disease panic! Cleanliness and food safety are easy to implement, but you will find yourself seeking out gluten in unusual places.

In thoroughly cleaning a kitchen, I prefer to start up high and end low. (Don't forget to clean inside drawers and cabinets!) Soap and water are the basics you'll need.

If your kitchen is not already dedicated gluten-free, I strongly suggest taking the following steps before making gluten-free cookies:

1. Allow your kitchen to be free of traditional wheat baking for at least overnight. Any lingering flour dust must settle and be cleaned away.

2. Remove all the items from the entire work area, including the sink, and wash your dedicated work area well. This would be a good time to be sure you wear a fresh apron (if your old one was used for baking with wheat). Don't forget fresh towels and potholders, too!

3. Thoroughly wash the mixer and beaters.

4. Gather nonporous utensils, bowls, measuring spoons and cups, and baking sheets. Wood and scratched plastic may harbor tiny gluten-particles—don't forget the rolling pin! (Nonstick surfaces are controversial as they can become scratched and cross-contaminated; it is better to just avoid them.) Wash all of these items well. Kitchen drawers are notorious for hiding food crumbs—clean them out and wipe them down. Storage containers should also be washed well.

5. Gather the ingredients for your recipe. All the ingredient packages should be unopened and free of any wayward traditional baking dust. (Note that just a little wayward traditional flour on a measuring cup or spoon can easily cross-contaminate other ingredients. A separate, safe storage area should be made for *all* ingredients used in gluten-free baking!) Also consider purchasing parchment paper. It is good to use on baking sheets (and cooling racks) to avoid potential cross-contamination from prior use with gluten-containing foods.

6. If in doubt about whether an ingredient is gluten-free, do not proceed! Read all ingredient labels carefully or call the manufacturer if you are unsure. Wheat should be clearly disclosed on any ingredient label in the United States.

7. Do not make any gluten-containing foods in the kitchen area until the cookies are packaged away. This is especially critical for flour dust! It travels despite the best of intentions.

The Cookie Pantry

Flours. With the exception of cornstarch and oats, all flours utilized in this book have been tested using Bob's Red Mill brand. These and similar high-quality gluten-free flours are available in larger grocery stores, online, and in numerous health food stores. Oats and oat flour must be obtained from a safe source (see the Appendix, page 180).

Unfortunately, the growing and harvesting of most oats involve fields, mills, and/or transport trucks that are also used for wheat, rye, or barley. That cross-contamination makes most oats unsafe for the gluten-free diet.

Baking Powder. Rumford brand has been utilized in all recipes.

Baking Soda. Arm & Hammer brand has been utilized in testing all recipes in this book.

Cocoa Powder. Hershey's cocoa has been my brand of choice. I personally prefer it to the flavor of Nestlé's.

Cream Cheese. Philadelphia is my favorite brand.

Decorations. Be sure to read the labels on icings and sprinkles. While writing these recipes, I noticed for the first time that some icings sold in tubes contain wheat. Careful!

Eggs. Any brand, size large.

Fats. All the recipes have been tested using Crisco brand shortening, (any brand) canola oil, and (any brand) lightly salted butter. If you must substitute margarine for butter, it should contain 80 percent fat.

Milk. 2% milk is my preference, but any percentage should be fine.

Salt. Any brand. Iodized salt is sometimes avoided by people having the skin manifestation of celiac disease (dermatitis herpetiformis). If you have dermatitis herpetiformis, you may wish to discuss with your health-care provider whether to use iodized salt.

Spices, Flavorings, Extracts. When possible, I prefer to use extracts instead of artificial flavorings. In any case, McCormick is my preferred brand. This company has a reputation for clearly labeling its product ingredients.

Sweeteners. White, brown, and confectioners' sugars: generally speaking, any brand is fine. However, confectioners' sugar is usually processed with cornstarch. Although unlikely, it is worth double-checking to be sure that wheat doesn't appear on the ingredient listing. Honey and molasses: any brand is generally fine.

Yogurt. Low-fat plain yogurt was used in testing these recipes. I avoid nonfat yogurt as the resultant cookies seem a bit off to me.

Equipment

Below is a list of the equipment I use in my kitchen. Most of my things are name brand but affordable. And as a side note, I highly recommend giving a baking-themed gift to anyone who has been diagnosed with dietary restrictions. A new rolling pin and a great sugar cookie recipe . . . a pizzelle iron and a bag of coffee . . . new spatulas and a bag of xanthan gum . . . all would touch the spirit.

Baking Pans and Sheets. I use aluminum or stainless steel baking pans and sheets. These are widely available in kitchen supply houses, craft stores, larger cooking departments, and kitchen specialty stores. I avoid nonstick surfaces, as they can become scratched and cross-contaminated. Nonstick cooking spray is ideal for lightly greasing the pans. Parchment paper works well with cookies and safeguards against cross-contamination from pans (especially nonstick) previously used for gluten-containing foods.

Blender. A blender is used in just a few recipes in this book (such as Fig Newton–Style Cookies, page 97). A handheld stick blender is ideal for this purpose. My Farberware model is now several years old and does a great job.

Cooling Racks. Any brand is fine. Be sure to cover the cooling racks with foil or parchment if they have been used previously for cooling gluten-containing foods. There are so may little nooks and crannies where cross-contamination could be an issue.

Cutting Boards. My collection of cutting boards is mostly plastic. Wooden boards are highly suspect for cross-contamination and should not be used (unless dedicated to only gluten-free use). Plastic boards with scratches may be suspect as well.

Measuring Spoons and Cups. Any name-brand measuring spoons and measuring cups are fine. I prefer metal measuring spoons and cups for durability and ease of cleaning. I use a Pyrex glass measuring cup. You may wish to avoid any plastic utensils (that have been previously used with gluten-containing foods) with scratches, due to possible cross-contamination.

Microwave Oven. Any brand. A microwave needs to be very, very clean! It is ideal for melting chocolates and making rice cereal bar cookies. Be sure to use microwave-safe bowls, cups, and pans; Pyrex is an ideal brand.

Mixer. I use a KitchenAid stand mixer. However, any strong hand mixer should work well with the recipes in this book. Also, nearly all of these recipes would do just fine mixed by hand.

Mixing Bowls. I use the large metal mixing bowl that came with my KitchenAid mixer. Metal and glass bowls are preferred for durability and ease of cleaning. You may wish to avoid any plastic bowls (used with gluten-containing foods) with scratches, due to possible cross-contamination.

Rolling Pin. I use a wooden "French" rolling pin. There are no mechanics to this rolling pin. It is simply a tapered piece of wood. It is one of my favorite kitchen tools. This rolling pin should be dedicated to gluten-free baking or covered with foil if previously used with gluten-containing doughs.

Scale. I use a Pelouze postage scale. Baking by weight is more accurate and faster. If using a scale, you will rarely need a measuring cup, as this scale (and now many others on the market) allow you to zero-out the weight of the bowl and weigh anew with each ingredient. The recipes in this book include weight measurements for dry ingredients.

School Supplies. A simple ruler and kitchen scissors come in handy again and again.

Specialty Items. Rosette irons, pizzelle makers, mini cookie cutters, etc. All of these items are available in larger cooking departments or kitchen specialty stores.

Utensils. Any brands and materials are fine as long as they are dedicated to gluten-free cooking only. Do not use wooden utensils, as these may be cross-contaminated. Spatulas can hide bits of gluten where the head meets the handle. Thorough cleaning or replacement is essential to avoid cross-contamination.

3

Drop Cookies

Drop cookies are at the heart of any cookie platter. They are quick to make and their flavors and textures vary tremendously. On occasion we all fall back on our longtime favorites, like Chocolate Chip or Oatmeal Raisin, and with good cause—they are delicious! However, I hope this chapter will expand your drop cookie repertoire. Perhaps you will be tempted by the soft and tender Almond Flower Cookies garnished with a splay of sliced almonds. Perhaps you'll make Coconut Macaroons. Or perhaps you will enjoy one of my new favorites, Lemon–Poppy Seed Cookies.

No matter which drop cookie you choose first, I trust you will be rewarded with oohs and aahs for your effort.

Almond Flower Cookies

brown rice flour and almond meal
MAKES ABOUT 25 COOKIES

This traditional version has sliced almonds arranged on top to resemble flowers.
These cookies are soft and moist.

$^1/_3$ cup oil, 65 grams

$^1/_2$ cup sugar, 100 grams

1 cup brown rice flour, 125 grams

2 eggs

$^1/_2$ cup almond meal, 60 grams

$^1/_4$ teaspoon baking soda

1 teaspoon baking powder

$^1/_2$ teaspoon salt

1 teaspoon xanthan gum

1 teaspoon almond extract

TOPPING (OPTIONAL):
$^1/_4$ cup sliced almonds

Preheat the oven to 350°F. Lightly grease a cookie sheet.

In a medium-size bowl, combine the oil and sugar. Beat well. Add the brown rice flour and beat well. Scrape down the sides of the mixing bowl at least once during mixing. Add the remaining ingredients and mix well.

Drop rounded teaspoonfuls of the dough onto the prepared pan. With moistened fingertips, press them to $^1/_4$-inch thickness. Arrange the almond slices on top into a flower or other nice pattern.

Bake the cookies for 8 to 10 minutes, until there is the slightest hint of color; the tops will be dry. Let cool on wire racks before serving.

Applesauce-Raisin Cookies

brown rice flour
MAKES ABOUT 40 COOKIES

It is such fun to have great ingredients in a tasty cookie. No guilt here!
Light in flavor and texture, they are sure to please.

$^1/_3$ cup oil, 65 grams

$^1/_2$ cup sugar, 100 grams

1$^1/_2$ cups brown rice flour,
185 grams

1 egg

$^1/_2$ cup applesauce

$^1/_4$ teaspoon baking soda

1 teaspoon baking powder

$^1/_2$ teaspoon salt

$^3/_4$ teaspoon xanthan gum

$^1/_4$ teaspoon vanilla extract
(optional)

$^1/_2$ teaspoon ground cinnamon

$^1/_3$ cup roughly chopped raisins,
55 grams

Preheat the oven to 350°F. Very lightly grease a cookie sheet.

In a medium-size bowl, combine the oil and sugar. Beat well. Add the flour and beat well. Scrape down the sides of the mixing bowl at least once during mixing. Add the remaining ingredients and beat well. Continue beating until the dough comes together; it will be soft.

Drop rounded teaspoonfuls of the dough onto the prepared pan. With moistened fingertips, press them to $^1/_4$-inch thickness.

Bake the cookies for about 10 minutes, until the edges begin to brown. Let cool on wire racks before serving.

Banana-Nut Cookies

brown rice flour

MAKES ABOUT 40 COOKIES

Inspired by one of my family's favorite snacks . . . banana bread.
These cookies are an understated treat.

⅓ cup oil, 65 grams

½ cup sugar, 100 grams

1½ cups brown rice flour,
    185 grams

1 egg

1 (4-ounce) jar Beech-Nut baby
    food bananas (stage 2),
    105 grams

¼ teaspoon baking soda

1 teaspoon baking powder

½ teaspoon salt

1¼ teaspoons xanthan gum

½ teaspoon vanilla extract

½ cup chopped pecans,
    60 grams

Preheat the oven to 350°F. Very lightly grease a cookie sheet.

In a medium-size bowl, combine the oil and sugar. Beat well. Add the flour and beat well. Add the remaining ingredients and beat well. Scrape down the sides of the mixing bowl at least once during mixing. Continue beating until the dough comes together; it will be soft.

Drop rounded teaspoonfuls of the dough onto the prepared pan. With moistened fingertips, press them to ¼-inch thickness. The cookies will hold this shape during baking, so you can place the cookies close together on the pan.

Bake the cookies for about 10 minutes, until the edges begin to brown. Let cool on wire racks before serving.

Chocolate Cookies with White Chips

brown rice flour

MAKES ABOUT 35 COOKIES

This cookie is the reverse of a chocolate chip cookie. It has the slightly drier texture of a store-bought cookie. It's perfect with a cup of tea or glass of milk.

$1/_3$ cup oil, 65 grams

$1/_2$ cup sugar, 100 grams

1 cup brown rice flour, 125 grams

$1/_4$ cup unsweetened cocoa powder, 20 grams

2 eggs

$1/_4$ teaspoon baking soda

1 teaspoon baking powder

$1/_2$ teaspoon salt

$1/_2$ teaspoon xanthan gum

1 teaspoon vanilla extract

$3/_4$ cup white chocolate chips, 130 grams

Preheat the oven to 350°F. Lightly grease a cookie sheet.

In a medium-size bowl, combine the oil and sugar. Beat well. Add the flour and beat well. Scrape down the sides of the mixing bowl at least once during mixing. Add the remaining ingredients and beat well. Continue beating until the dough comes together. The dough will be very soft and a little sticky.

Drop rounded teaspoonfuls of the dough onto the prepared pan. With moistened fingertips, press them to 1/4-inch thickness.

Bake the cookies for about 9 minutes, until the tops are dry. Let cool on wire racks before serving.

Chocolate Chip Cookies #1

brown rice flour and cornstarch
MAKES ABOUT 30 COOKIES

A really tasty chocolate chip cookie!
Enjoy them hot from the oven . . . what a treat!

$^1/_3$ cup oil, 65 grams

$^1/_2$ cup brown sugar (dark if possible), 100 grams

1 cup brown rice flour, 125 grams

$^1/_3$ cup cornstarch, 40 grams

2 eggs

$^1/_4$ teaspoon baking soda

$^1/_2$ teaspoon salt

$^3/_4$ teaspoon xanthan gum

1 teaspoon vanilla extract

1 cup semisweet chocolate chips, 160 grams

Preheat the oven to 350°F. Lightly grease a cookie sheet.

In a medium-size bowl, combine the oil and sugar. Beat well. Add the brown rice flour and cornstarch and beat well. Scrape down the sides of the mixing bowl at least once during mixing. Add the remaining ingredients, except for the chocolate chips, and mix well. Stir in the chocolate chips.

Drop rounded teaspoonfuls of the dough onto the prepared pan. With moistened fingertips, press them to $^1/_4$-inch thickness, for a better cookie shape. Bake the cookies for about 10 minutes, until the edges begin to brown. Let cool on wire racks before serving.

Chocolate Chip Cookies #2

sorghum flour

MAKES ABOUT 24 COOKIES

Unlike most chocolate chip cookies, this recipe calls for regular sugar instead of brown sugar. The whole-grain taste of the sorghum does a fabulous job in making these cookies taste just right.

$^1/_3$ cup oil, 65 grams

2 tablespoons butter

$^1/_2$ cup sugar, 100 grams

1 cup sorghum flour, 135 grams

1 egg

$^1/_4$ teaspoon baking soda

$^1/_2$ teaspoon salt

1 teaspoon xanthan gum

1 teaspoon vanilla extract

1 cup semisweet chocolate chips, 160 grams

Preheat the oven to 350°F. Lightly grease a cookie sheet.

In a medium-size bowl, combine the oil, butter, and sugar. Beat well. Add the sorghum flour and beat well. Scrape down the sides of the mixing bowl at least once during mixing. Add the remaining ingredients and mix well. Continue beating until the dough comes together. The dough will be soft and seem oily.

Drop rounded teaspoonfuls of the dough onto the prepared pan. With moistened fingertips, press them to $^1/_4$-inch thickness.

Bake the cookies for 8 to 10 minutes, until the edges are lightly browned. Let cool on wire racks before serving.

Coconut Macaroons

brown rice flour

MAKES ABOUT 20 COOKIES

This recipe is an adaptation of the Coconut Macaroons recipe on the back of the Baker's Angel Flake Coconut bag. I don't want you to miss out on this tasty cookie when making them is so easy! If you are substituting another brand of coconut, please note that this coconut is sweetened.

1 (7-ounce) package sweetened flaked coconut (2 2/3 cups)

1/3 cup sugar, 75 grams

2 tablespoons brown rice flour

Pinch of salt (scant 1/8 teaspoon)

Pinch of xanthan gum (scant 1/8 teaspoon)

2 egg whites

1/2 teaspoon vanilla or almond extract

Preheat the oven to 350°F. Lightly grease a cookie sheet.

In a medium-size bowl, combine all the ingredients in the order given. Beat well. The mixture will look like loose, moistened coconut. Drop rounded teaspoonfuls of the dough onto the prepared pan.

Bake the cookies for 15 to 20 minutes, until the edges are golden brown. Let cool on wire racks before serving.

Cranberry Cookies

sorghum flour

MAKES ABOUT 24 COOKIES

These cookies are inspired by a Girl Scout favorite,
Thank U Berry Munch. The gluten-free version produces tender,
understated cookies with a hint of whole-grain flavor.

$1/3$ cup oil, 65 grams

2 tablespoons butter

$1/2$ cup sugar, 100 grams

1 cup sorghum flour, 135 grams

1 egg

$1/4$ teaspoon baking soda

$1/2$ teaspoon salt

1 teaspoon xanthan gum

$1^{1}/_{2}$ teaspoons vanilla extract

$1/3$ cup finely chopped dried
sweetened cranberries,
40 grams

Preheat the oven to 350°F. Lightly grease a
cookie sheet.

In a medium-size bowl, combine the oil, butter,
and sugar. Beat well. Add the sorghum flour
and beat well. Scrape down the sides of the
mixing bowl at least once during mixing.
Add the remaining ingredients and mix well.
Continue beating until the dough comes together. The dough will be soft and seem oily.

Drop rounded teaspoonfuls of the dough onto
the prepared pan. With moistened fingertips,
flatten them to $1/4$-inch thickness.

Bake the cookies for 8 to 10 minutes, until the
edges are lightly browned. Let cool on wire
racks before serving.

Ginger Spice Cookies

sorghum flour

MAKES ABOUT 24 COOKIES

These cookies are tender and spicy, yet mellowed by a bit of vanilla flavoring. Omit the vanilla for more "bite."

$1/3$ cup oil, 65 grams

$1/2$ cup brown sugar, 100 grams

1 cup sorghum flour, 135 grams

1 egg

$1/4$ teaspoon baking soda

$1/2$ teaspoon salt

1 teaspoon xanthan gum

1 teaspoon ground ginger

$1^1/_2$ teaspoons pumpkin pie spice

$1/4$ teaspoon vanilla extract

TOPPING:
2 tablespoons sugar

Preheat the oven to 350°F. Lightly grease a cookie sheet.

In a medium-size bowl, combine the oil and sugar. Beat well. Add the sorghum flour and beat well. Scrape down the sides of the mixing bowl at least once during mixing. Add the remaining ingredients and mix well. Continue beating until the dough comes together. The dough will look like a traditional cookie dough.

Drop rounded teaspoonfuls of the dough onto the prepared pan. For the topping, place the 2 tablespoons of sugar in a bowl. Dip the bottom of a glass into water to moisten it, then dip it into the sugar. Use the sugared glass to press the dough balls to $1/8$- to $1/4$-inch thickness.

Bake the cookies for 8 minutes, until they just begin to brown at the edges. These cookies will crisp a little during cooling. Let cool on wire racks before serving.

Hermits

sorghum flour

MAKES ABOUT 24 COOKIES

A classic combination of coffee, spices, raisins, and nuts.

⅓ cup oil, 65 grams

½ cup brown sugar, 100 grams

1 cup sorghum flour, 135 grams

1 egg

¼ teaspoon baking soda

½ teaspoon salt

1 teaspoon xanthan gum

1½ teaspoons pumpkin pie spice

1½ teaspoons instant coffee
dissolved in 1 teaspoon water

¼ teaspoon vanilla extract

½ cup raisins, 80 grams

½ cup chopped pecans,
60 grams

TOPPING (OPTIONAL):
2 tablespoons confectioners'
sugar

Preheat the oven to 350°F. Lightly grease a cookie sheet.

In a medium-size bowl, combine the oil and sugar. Beat well. Add the sorghum flour and beat well. Scrape down the sides of the mixing bowl at least once during mixing. Add the remaining ingredients and mix well. Continue beating until the dough comes together. The dough will look like a traditional cookie dough.

Drop rounded teaspoonfuls of the dough onto the prepared pan. With moist fingertips, press them to ⅛- to ¼-inch thickness.

Bake the cookies for 8 minutes, until they just begin to brown at the edges. The cookies will crisp a little during cooling. Let cool on wire racks before serving.

Dust the tops of the cookies with confectioners' sugar if desired.

Hot Chocolate Cookies

brown rice flour

MAKES ABOUT 30 COOKIES

This cookie tastes like hot chocolate with tiny marshmallows melted on top. I hope you enjoy these as much as I enjoyed creating them. They are slightly crisp on the outside and soft inside.

$1/3$ cup oil, 65 grams

$1/2$ cup sugar, 100 grams

$1 1/4$ cups brown rice flour, 155 grams

1 egg

$1/2$ cup chocolate syrup (such as Hershey's)

$1/4$ teaspoon baking soda

2 teaspoons baking powder

$1/2$ teaspoon salt

1 teaspoon xanthan gum

1 teaspoon vanilla extract

$1/3$ cup finely chopped mini marshmallows

Preheat the oven to 350°F. Very lightly grease a cookie sheet.

In a medium-size bowl, combine the oil and sugar. Beat well. Add the brown rice flour and beat well. Scrape down the sides of the mixing bowl at least once during mixing. Add the remaining ingredients, except the marshmallows, and beat well. Continue beating until the dough comes together; it will be soft and sticky. Gently mix in the marshmallows.

Drop rounded teaspoonfuls of the dough onto the prepared pan.

Bake the cookies for about 9 minutes, until the edges begin to brown. Let cool for a minute or so on the baking sheet to make the cookies easier to remove. (The cookies will flatten during cooling.) Let cool on wire racks before serving.

Lace Cookies, Oatmeal

oats

MAKES ABOUT 20 COOKIES

Suggested by my good friend Theresa, I've included these tasty cookies! This dough will spread into a lacy, crisp cookie. If you work quickly, you can shape them into tubes. If not, enjoy them flat. Although not traditional, I've included a bit of vanilla to soften the flavor of this cookie.

1¼ cups rolled oats, 125 grams

⅓ cup oil, 65 grams

½ cup brown sugar, 100 grams

1 egg

¼ teaspoon salt

1 teaspoon baking powder

Pinch of xanthan gum

½ teaspoon vanilla extract

Preheat the oven to 350°F. Liberally grease a cookie sheet or a sheet of foil placed on the cookie sheet.

Place the oatmeal in a blender. Process until a third of the oatmeal is powdery; the rest may be of varying sizes.

Pour the oatmeal into a mixing bowl. Add the remaining ingredients and mix very well. A sticky-looking dough will form.

Place the dough by the tablespoonful onto the prepared pan. With moist fingertips, press the dough to ⅛-inch thickness.

Bake the cookies for 6 to 9 minutes, until they are lightly browned and appear cooked in the center. Keep the cookies on the pan for a minute or two to set. Gently ease the cookies from the cookie sheet with a spatula. The cookies will be pliable, yet have real substance. Let cool on wire racks before serving.

Lemon-Poppy Seed Cookies

brown rice flour
MAKES ABOUT 30 COOKIES

These cookies are inspired by lemon–poppy seed pound cake. A delicate cookie full of poppy seeds and topped with an exceptional lemon glaze.

$^1\!/_3$ cup oil, 65 grams

$^1\!/_2$ cup sugar, 100 grams

$1^1\!/_4$ cups brown rice flour, 155 grams

1 egg

$^1\!/_4$ teaspoon baking soda

1 teaspoon baking powder

$^1\!/_2$ teaspoon salt

1 teaspoon xanthan gum

2 tablespoons frozen lemonade concentrate

1 teaspoon lemon extract

1 tablespoon poppy seeds

TOPPING:

$^1\!/_2$ cup confectioners' sugar

2 tablespoons frozen lemonade concentrate

Preheat the oven to 350°F. Lightly grease a cookie sheet.

In a medium-size bowl, combine the oil and sugar. Beat well. Add the brown rice flour and beat well. Scrape down the sides of the mixing bowl at least once during mixing. Add the remaining ingredients and beat well. Continue beating until the dough comes together. The dough will be quite thick.

Drop rounded teaspoonfuls of the dough onto the prepared pan. With moistened fingertips, press them to $^1\!/_4$-inch thickness.

Bake the cookies for 8 to 10 minutes, until they are lightly browned at the edges. Let cool on wire racks. Mix the confectioners' sugar with the 2 tablespoons of frozen lemonade concentrate. Drizzle the topping over the cookies.

Molasses Cookies

brown rice flour

MAKES ABOUT 20 COOKIES

Soft, moist, and lightly spiced. A hint of glaze adds to this favorite cookie,
should you like them extra sweet.

$\frac{1}{3}$ cup oil, 65 grams

$\frac{1}{4}$ cup sugar, 50 grams

1$\frac{1}{2}$ cups brown rice flour,
185 grams

$\frac{1}{4}$ cup unsulfured molasses,
85 grams

1 egg

$\frac{1}{2}$ teaspoon baking soda

$\frac{1}{2}$ teaspoon salt

$\frac{1}{2}$ teaspoon xanthan gum

$\frac{1}{2}$ teaspoon pumpkin pie spice

$\frac{1}{2}$ cup raisins (optional),
80 grams

TOPPING (OPTIONAL):

1 cup confectioners' sugar

About 4 teaspoons milk

Preheat the oven to 350°F. Lightly grease a cookie sheet.

In a medium-size bowl, combine the oil and sugar. Beat well. Add the brown rice flour and beat well. Scrape down the sides of the mixing bowl at least once during mixing. Add the remaining ingredients and beat well. Continue beating until the dough is well blended.

Drop rounded tablespoonfuls of the dough onto the prepared pan. With moistened fingertips, press them to $\frac{1}{4}$-inch thickness.

Bake the cookies for about 10 minutes, until the edges begin to brown. Let cool on wire racks.

If desired, combine the topping ingredients to form a glaze and lightly ice the tops of the cookies.

Mrs. Fields- or Neiman Marcus-Style Cookies

sorghum flour and oats
MAKES ABOUT 36 COOKIES

Packed full of the good stuff you expect in these popular cookies. I chose to use pecans in this recipe because it is my favorite nut for baking, but use your favorite. Despite using healthy, whole grains, I cannot call these cookies healthy. They are decadent. I urge portion control!

1/3 cup oil, 65 grams

2 tablespoons butter

1/2 cup brown sugar, 100 grams

3/4 cup sorghum flour, 100 grams

1/2 cup rolled oats, pulsed in a blender to make smaller pieces of all sizes, 50 grams

1 egg

1/4 teaspoon baking soda

1/2 teaspoon salt

1 teaspoon xanthan gum

1 teaspoon vanilla extract

1/2 cup semisweet chocolate chips, 80 grams

1/2 cup chopped pecans, 50 grams

2 ounces milk chocolate (from a bar), grated (just over 1/2 cup)

Preheat the oven to 350°F. Lightly grease a cookie sheet.

In a medium-size bowl, combine the oil, butter, and sugar. Beat well. Add the sorghum flour and beat well. Scrape down the sides of the mixing bowl at least once during mixing. Add the remaining ingredients, except the chocolates and nuts, and mix well. Continue beating until the dough comes together. Mix in the chocolates and nuts. The dough will be soft and seem oily.

Drop rounded teaspoonfuls of the dough onto the prepared pan. With moistened fingertips, press them to 1/4- to 1/3-inch thickness.

Bake the cookies for 8 to 10 minutes, until the edges are lightly browned. Let cool on wire racks before serving.

Oatmeal-Raisin Cookies

brown rice flour

MAKES ABOUT 30 COOKIES

Rather than having you purchase individual spices for "spiced" cookies in this book, I have opted for pumpkin pie spice, saving space and budget.

$1/3$ cup oil, 65 grams

$1/2$ cup brown sugar, 100 grams

$1\frac{1}{2}$ cups brown rice flour, 185 grams

$1/2$ cup rolled oats, pulsed in a blender to make smaller pieces, 50 grams

$1/2$ cup raisins, 80 grams

1 egg

$1/4$ teaspoon baking soda

$1/2$ teaspoon salt

$3/4$ teaspoon xanthan gum

$1/2$ teaspoon vanilla extract (optional)

1 teaspoon pumpkin pie spice

3 tablespoons water

TOPPING (OPTIONAL):

$1/2$ cup confectioners' sugar

About 2 teaspoons milk

Preheat the oven to 350°F. Lightly grease a cookie sheet.

In a medium-size bowl, combine the oil and sugar. Beat well. Add the brown rice flour and beat well. Scrape down the sides of the mixing bowl at least once during mixing. Add the remaining ingredients and beat well. Continue beating until the dough comes together.

Drop rounded teaspoonfuls of the dough onto the prepared pan. With moistened fingertips, press them to $1/4$-inch thickness.

Bake the cookies for about 10 minutes, until the edges begin to brown. Let cool on wire racks.

If desired, combine the topping ingredients to form a glaze. Drizzle it over the tops of the cookies.

Peanut Butter Blossom Cookies

brown rice flour and cornstarch

MAKES ABOUT 26 COOKIES

A classic peanut butter cookie with a milk chocolate kiss right in the middle. The cookie has a light tenderness to it that blends perfectly with the understated milk chocolate flavor.

¼ cup creamy peanut butter, 65 grams

2 tablespoons oil, 20 grams

½ cup brown sugar, 100 grams

1 cup brown rice flour, 125 grams

⅓ cup cornstarch, 40 grams

1 egg

¼ teaspoon baking soda

1 teaspoon baking powder

½ teaspoon salt

1 teaspoon xanthan gum

1 teaspoon vanilla extract

2 tablespoons water

TOPPING:
1 to 2 tablespoons sugar

26 milk chocolate kisses

Preheat the oven to 350°F. Lightly grease a cookie sheet.

In a medium-size bowl, combine the peanut butter, oil, and sugar. Beat well. Add the brown rice flour and cornstarch and beat well. Scrape down the sides of the mixing bowl at least once during mixing. Add the remaining ingredients and beat well. Continue beating until the dough comes together.

Shape the dough into 1-inch balls. Roll them in sugar and place them on the prepared pan. Press the tops to flatten them slightly.

Bake the cookies for 10 to 12 minutes, until the edges begin to have a hint of browning. Remove the sheet from the oven. Immediately press a chocolate kiss into the center of each cookie. Let cool on wire racks before serving.

Pecan Cookies

brown rice flour
MAKES ABOUT 30 COOKIES

Whereas a Pecan Sandie is a dry, tender cookie, this is a soft, tender cookie.

⅓ cup shortening, 70 grams

½ cup brown sugar, 100 grams

1 cup brown rice flour, 125 grams

1 egg, plus 1 egg yolk

½ cup pecan meal, 40 grams

¼ teaspoon baking soda

½ teaspoon baking powder

½ teaspoon salt

1 teaspoon xanthan gum

1 teaspoon vanilla extract

Preheat the oven to 350°F. Lightly grease a baking sheet.

In a medium-size bowl, combine the shortening and sugar. Beat well. Add the brown rice flour and beat well. Scrape down the sides of the mixing bowl at least once during mixing. Add the remaining ingredients and mix well; the dough will be quite thick.

Drop rounded teaspoonfuls of the dough onto the prepared pan.

Bake the cookies for 8 to 10 minutes, until there is the slightest hint of color; the tops of the cookies will be dry. Let cool on wire racks before serving.

Pecan Lace Cookies

pecan meal

MAKES ABOUT 20 COOKIES

A delicate version of lace cookies. They are delicious, bright, crisp on the edges, and almost nougatlike in the middle. Their appearance is more like a wafer than a lace cookie.

³/₄ cup finely chopped pecans, 85 grams

¹/₄ cup pecan meal (flour), 20 grams

¹/₃ cup oil, 65 grams

¹/₂ cup brown sugar, 100 grams

2 eggs

¹/₄ teaspoon salt

Pinch of xanthan gum

1 teaspoon vanilla extract

Preheat the oven to 350°F. Grease a cookie sheet very well.

Combine all the ingredients and mix very well. The dough will need a few minutes of beating to develop body; this is important. As you beat the mixture, it will first look like a thick table syrup, then, with continued beating, a sticky-looking dough will form.

Place the dough by the tablespoonful onto the prepared pan. With moistened fingertips, press the dough to a scant ⅛-inch thickness.

Bake the cookies for 6 to 9 minutes, until they are lightly browned and appear cooked in the center. Keep the cookies on the pan for a minute or two to "set." Gently ease them from the cookie sheet with a spatula. The cookies will be pliable, yet have real substance. Let cool on wire racks before serving.

Note: If you have trouble finding pecan meal, you can grind pecans (with brief pulses) in a blender or coffee mill to a flourlike consistency.

Sour Cream Breakfast Cookies

brown rice flour

MAKES ABOUT 35 COOKIES

Inspired by that great breakfast coffee cake, these cookies are a terrific excuse for eating breakfast on the run! They are rich, moist, and flavorful.

1/3 cup oil, 65 grams

1/2 cup sugar, 100 grams

1 1/2 cups brown rice flour, 185 grams

1 egg

1/2 cup sour cream

1/4 teaspoon baking soda

1 teaspoon baking powder

1/2 teaspoon salt

3/4 teaspoon xanthan gum

1 teaspoon vanilla extract

TOPPING:

3 tablespoons brown sugar

1/2 teaspoon ground cinnamon

2 tablespoons butter, 30 grams

Preheat the oven to 350°F. Very lightly grease a cookie sheet.

In a medium-size bowl, combine the oil and sugar. Beat well. Add the flour and beat well. Scrape down the sides of the mixing bowl at least once during mixing. Add the remaining cookie ingredients and beat well. Continue beating until the dough comes together; it will be soft. Set aside.

In a separate bowl, mix together the brown sugar, cinnamon, and butter to form a crumble. (If the butter is soft, the crumble may not crumble at all. This is okay.) Set aside.

Drop rounded teaspoonfuls of the dough onto the prepared pan. With moistened fingertips, press them to 1/4-inch thickness. Place a small amount of crumble mixture on top of each cookie.

Bake the cookies for about 10 minutes, until the edges begin to brown. Let cool on wire racks before serving.

Note: You may be tempted to just fold the topping crumble mixture into the dough mixture. Unfortunately, this creates areas where the topping will run onto the baking sheet. Adding the topping as directed will give you the desired result.

4

Bar Cookies

Are you ever in a hurry for something wonderful? This chapter is full of delicious bar cookies. While I am a huge fan of any cookie dark with chocolate (such as my Decadent Brownies!), three of my favorites in this chapter are Carrot Cake Bars, Jam Bars, and White Chocolate Bars. And if you are in a super hurry, try either version of the Rice Cereal Bars. Sure, they are traditionally fast to make in the first place, but you can microwave the marshmallow mixture in just two minutes! Not even a messy pot to clean. I've topped the traditional version with just a little chocolate . . . which makes it so much better than you can imagine.

I used to be in a rut, making just one or two favorite bar cookies, but not anymore. I hope you find new favorites here, too.

Almond Layered Cookie Bars

brown rice flour and almond meal

MAKES 15 COOKIES

A tasty cookie bar full of good stuff! Let the bar cool fully to allow the structure to set. Then enjoy the multitude of tempting layers!

½ cup butter, 110 grams

½ cup sugar, 100 grams

1 cup brown rice flour, 125 grams

1 egg

½ cup almond meal, 60 grams

¼ teaspoon baking soda

2 teaspoons baking powder

½ teaspoon salt

1 teaspoon xanthan gum

1 teaspoon vanilla extract

TOPPING:
1 (14-ounce) can sweetened condensed milk

1 cup sweetened flaked coconut, 120 grams

1 (4-ounce) package sliced almonds

1½ cups chocolate chips, 240 grams

Preheat the oven to 350°F. Lightly grease an 8-inch square baking pan.

In a medium-size bowl, combine the butter and sugar. Beat well. Add the brown rice flour and continue to beat well. Add the remaining dough ingredients and mix well. The cookie dough will be heavy.

Press the dough evenly into the bottom of the prepared pan. Bake for about 15 minutes, until golden brown. Layer with the condensed milk, coconut, almonds, and chocolate chips, and bake for an additional 25 minutes. The toppings will take on a bit of color.

Let cool completely and cut into bars.

Apple Crumble Bars

brown rice flour

MAKES 15 COOKIES

This cookie bar is fashioned after those found in a little bakery in Shepherdstown, West Virginia, a pretty college town near my home that is peppered with quaint restaurants. Although not called for in the recipe, a few tablespoons of finely chopped raisins would be a very nice addition to the topping. These cookies are sweet!

$^1/_3$ cup oil, 65 grams

$^1/_2$ cup sugar, 100 grams

1$^1/_4$ cups brown rice flour, 155 grams

1 egg

$^1/_4$ teaspoon baking soda

1 teaspoon baking powder

$^1/_2$ teaspoon salt

1 teaspoon xanthan gum

1 tablespoon water

1 teaspoon vanilla extract

$^1/_2$ teaspoon ground cinnamon

TOPPING:

1 apple (a sweet variety such as Gala or Golden Delicious), peeled and diced small (about 1 cup)

$^1/_4$ cup sugar

$^1/_4$ cup water

1$^1/_2$ teaspoons cornstarch or potato starch

$^1/_4$ teaspoon ground cinnamon

$^1/_3$ of dough reserved from above (135 grams)

Preheat the oven to 350°F. Lightly grease an 8-inch square baking pan.

In a medium-size bowl, combine the oil and sugar. Beat well. Add the brown rice flour and beat well. Scrape down the sides of the mixing bowl at least once during mixing. Add the remaining dough ingredients and beat well. Continue beating until the dough comes together; it will be quite thick.

Press two-thirds of the dough evenly into the prepared pan. Set aside.

In a microwave-safe bowl, combine all the topping ingredients, except the retained dough. Stir well. Microwave on HIGH for about 2 minutes, until the apples are soft and the sauce is clear and thick. Stir and check the topping after 1 minute. Spread the mixture over the top of the dough in the pan.

Top with bits of the remaining dough. (It should look crumbly.) Bake for 20 to 25 minutes, until lightly browned and a toothpick tests cleanly. Let cool before slicing and serving.

Blondies #1

brown rice flour

MAKES 15 COOKIES

*This cookie is great even without the chocolate topping,
but I just couldn't resist.*

$\frac{1}{3}$ cup oil, 65 grams

$\frac{1}{2}$ cup brown sugar, 100 grams

1$\frac{1}{4}$ cups brown rice flour,
   155 grams

1 egg

$\frac{1}{4}$ teaspoon baking soda

1 teaspoon baking powder

$\frac{1}{2}$ teaspoon salt

1 teaspoon xanthan gum

2 tablespoons water

1 teaspoon vanilla extract

$\frac{1}{2}$ cup chopped pecans,
   60 grams

TOPPING:
$\frac{2}{3}$ cup mini chocolate chips,
   60 grams

Preheat the oven to 350°F. Lightly grease an 8-inch square baking pan.

In a medium-size bowl, combine the oil and sugar. Beat well. Add the brown rice flour and beat well. Scrape down the sides of the mixing bowl at least once during mixing. Add the remaining dough ingredients and beat well. Continue beating until the dough comes together; it will be quite thick.

Press the dough evenly into the prepared pan. Bake for about 20 minutes, until lightly browned and a toothpick tests cleanly.

While still hot, spread the chocolate chips over the top and cover with foil or a baking sheet. When the chocolate is melted, spread it across the tops of bars to coat evenly. Let cool completely and cut into bars.

Blondies #2

sorghum flour
MAKES 18 COOKIES

A dense, moist, brownielike bar with nuts, but not chocolate. I do include a little melted chocolate to drizzle over the tops, but you may resist if you like. These cookies are delicious at room temperature, but not as much when warm.

1/3 cup oil, 65 grams

2 tablespoons butter

1/2 cup brown sugar, 100 grams

1 cup sorghum flour, 135 grams

1/2 cup chopped pecans or other nuts, 60 grams

2 eggs

1/4 teaspoon baking soda

1/2 teaspoon salt

3/4 teaspoon xanthan gum

1 teaspoon vanilla extract

TOPPING:
2 ounces semisweet or milk chocolate, melted

Preheat the oven to 350°F. Lightly grease an 8-inch square baking pan.

In a medium-size bowl, combine the oil, butter, and sugar. Beat well. Add the sorghum flour and beat well. Scrape down the sides of the mixing bowl at least once during mixing. Add the remaining ingredients and mix well. Continue beating until the dough comes together; it will be a heavy batter.

Spread the dough evenly in the prepared pan. Bake for 20 minutes, until a toothpick tests cleanly and the edges begin to brown (and pull away from the sides of the pan).

Let cool. Cut into 18 bars. Drizzle melted chocolate over the top of the bars, if desired.

Carrot Cake Bars

brown rice flour

MAKES 15 COOKIES

This cookie bar has carrots, raisins, and nuts. I like these cookies without the frosting, but have included a little cream cheese icing if you want to be spoiled! By combining shortening with the cream cheese, the sticky sweetness of traditional icing is avoided.

1/3 cup oil, 65 grams

1/2 cup sugar, 100 grams

1 1/4 cups brown rice flour, 155 grams

1 egg, plus 1 egg yolk

1/4 teaspoon baking soda

2 teaspoons baking powder

1/2 teaspoon salt

1 teaspoon xanthan gum

1 teaspoon vanilla extract

1 1/2 teaspoons pumpkin pie spice

1/2 cup packed grated carrots, 75 grams

1/2 cup raisins, 80 grams

1/2 cup chopped walnuts, 35 grams

ICING:

2 tablespoons shortening, 25 grams

1/2 cup confectioners' sugar, 60 grams

3 ounces cream cheese, 85 grams

1/4 teaspoon vanilla extract

Preheat the oven to 350°F. Lightly grease an 8-inch square baking pan.

In a medium-size bowl, combine the oil and sugar. Beat well. Add the brown rice flour and beat well. Scrape down the sides of the mixing bowl at least once during mixing. Add the remaining dough ingredients and beat well. Continue beating until the dough comes together; it will be quite thick.

Press the dough evenly into the prepared pan. Bake for 20 to 25 minutes, until lightly browned and a toothpick tests cleanly. Let cool.

To make the icing, mix the icing ingredients until well blended. Spread over the cookies. Cut into bars.

Cheesecake Bars

brown rice flour
MAKES 15 COOKIES

Enjoy these rich bars in small proportion! They have the richness of cheesecake crossed with the tender crumb of a cookie.

1/3 cup shortening, 70 grams

1/2 cup sugar, 100 grams

2 egg whites

1 1/2 cups brown rice flour, 185 grams

1/2 teaspoon salt

1/4 teaspoon baking soda

2 teaspoons baking powder

1 teaspoon xanthan gum

1/2 teaspoon vanilla extract

TOPPING:
1 (8-ounce) package cream cheese

1/3 cup softened butter, 70 grams

1 1/4 cups confectioners' sugar, 150 grams

1 egg

1/2 teaspoon vanilla extract

1/3 cup raspberry jam (or other favorite)

Preheat the oven to 350°F. Lightly grease an 8-inch square baking pan.

In a medium-size bowl, combine the shortening and sugar. Beat well. Add the flour and beat well. Scrape down the sides of the mixing bowl at least once during mixing. Add the remaining dough ingredients and mix well until the dough comes together.

Press the dough evenly into the prepared pan. Bake for 5 minutes, then set aside. Reduce the heat to 325°F.

In a small bowl, combine the topping ingredients, except the jam. Beat until creamy. Pour the topping over the cookie dough. Stir the jam to make it easier to spread and scatter tablespoons of jam over the topping. Using a knife, swirl the jam through the topping.

Bake for about 45 minutes, until the top layer is lightly browned and set. Let cool completely and cut into bars.

Cranberry-Orange-Almond Granola Bars

oats and brown rice flour
MAKES 12 COOKIES

Inspired by my gluten-free friends, these granola bars are full of feel-good ingredients. Substitute your favorite dried fruits and nuts for mine. If it sounds good, it probably will be. Please note that these bars are like a soft, heavy oatmeal cookie when first baked. Let them mellow for a day or two and they are much better!

1/3 cup melted butter, 70 grams

1/2 cup honey, 160 grams

2 cups rolled oats, 160 grams

1/2 cup brown rice flour, 60 grams

1/4 teaspoon baking soda

1/2 teaspoon xanthan gum

1/2 cup chopped sweetened, dried cranberries, 50 grams

1/2 cup sliced almonds, 35 grams, toasted

1 tablespoon orange zest

Preheat the oven to 325°F. Lightly grease an 8-inch square baking pan.

In a large bowl, combine the butter and honey. Mix well. Add all the remaining ingredients and mix well. Pour the batter into the prepared pan and press firmly. Bake for 20 to 25 minutes until lightly browned. Let cool and cut into bars.

Notes: To toast sliced almonds, spray a small skillet with nonstick spray and heat to medium heat. Add the almonds and fry until lightly browned. Stir frequently and watch carefully to avoid burning the almonds. The almonds should be lightly browned and fragrant.

To make orange zest without a zester, just peel a bit of the outermost edge of an orange with a potato peeler. Then cut into very narrow strips, using a knife.

| The Ultimate Gluten-Free Cookie Book

Decadent Brownies

sorghum flour

MAKES 16 BROWNIES

A little cakey, a little gooey when warm, a little dense, and, oh so chocolaty. These are especially good warm from the oven. (I'm thinking brownie sundaes!)

¹/₃ cup oil, 65 grams

¹/₂ cup brown sugar, 100 grams

1 cup sorghum flour, 135 grams

¹/₃ cup unsweetened cocoa powder, 30 grams

2 eggs

¹/₄ teaspoon baking soda

1 teaspoon baking powder

¹/₂ teaspoon salt

³/₄ teaspoon xanthan gum

1 teaspoon vanilla extract

¹/₂ cup mini semisweet chocolate chips, 90 grams

TOPPING (OPTIONAL):
¹/₄ cup mini semisweet chocolate chips, 45 grams

Preheat the oven to 350°F. Lightly grease an 8-inch square baking pan.

In a medium-size bowl, combine the oil and sugar. Beat well. Add the sorghum flour and cocoa and beat well. Scrape down the sides of the mixing bowl at least once during mixing. Add the remaining ingredients and mix well. Continue beating until the dough comes together; it will be stiff and a little oily.

Press the dough evenly into the prepared pan. Bake for 15 minutes, until the cookie tests cleanly with a toothpick. If desired, immediately after removing the pan from the oven, sprinkle the mini chocolate chips over the brownies and cover with foil or a baking sheet. Once the chips melt, spread with a knife to form a very thin chocolate topping. Let cool completely and cut into bars.

Jam Bars

brown rice flour
MAKES 15 COOKIES

This cookie bar is so much easier to prepare than a Danish, while every bit as tasty. I use raspberry jam, but substitute your favorite for mine!

¹/₃ cup oil, 65 grams

¹/₂ cup sugar, 100 grams

1¹/₄ cups brown rice flour, 155 grams

1 egg

¹/₄ teaspoon baking soda

2 teaspoons baking powder

¹/₂ teaspoon salt

1 teaspoon xanthan gum

2 tablespoons water

1 teaspoon vanilla extract

TOPPING:
¹/₃ of dough reserved from above (135 grams)

¹/₂ cup seedless raspberry jam

2 tablespoons confectioners' sugar

Preheat the oven to 350°F. Lightly grease an 8-inch square baking pan.

In a medium-size bowl, combine the oil and sugar. Beat well. Add the brown rice flour and beat well. Scrape down the sides of the mixing bowl at least once during mixing. Add the remaining dough ingredients and beat well. Continue beating until the dough comes together; it will be quite thick.

Press two-thirds of the dough evenly into the prepared pan. Spread the jam over the dough and top with bits of the remaining dough. (I like to flatten the bits of dough between greased fingertips and lay them on top of the jam, much like for a cobbler.) Bake for 20 to 25 minutes, until lightly browned and a toothpick tests cleanly. Dust with confectioners' sugar. Let cool completely and cut into bars.

Lemon Bars

brown rice flour
MAKES 12 COOKIES

Lemon curd atop a lemon cookie base. Frozen lemonade concentrate provides fresh lemon flavor. Serving these with a garnish of lemon peel is very pretty.

¹/₃ cup oil, 65 grams

¹/₂ cup sugar, 100 grams

1¹/₄ cups brown rice flour, 155 grams

1 egg

¹/₄ teaspoon baking soda

1 teaspoon baking powder

¹/₂ teaspoon salt

1 teaspoon xanthan gum

2 tablespoons frozen lemonade concentrate

1 teaspoon lemon extract

TOPPING:

1 cup water

¹/₂ cup frozen lemonade concentrate

1 egg

¹/₄ cup cornstarch or potato starch, 35 grams

1 tablespoon confectioners' sugar

Preheat the oven to 350°F. Lightly grease an 8-inch square baking pan.

In a medium-size bowl, combine the oil and sugar. Beat well. Add the brown rice flour and beat well. Scrape down the sides of the mixing bowl at least once during mixing. Add the remaining batter ingredients and beat well. Continue beating until the dough comes together; it will be quite thick.

Press the dough evenly into the prepared pan. Bake for about 20 minutes, until lightly browned and a toothpick tests cleanly. Let cool.

In a microwave-safe cup, combine the topping ingredients, except for the confectioners' sugar, and mix well. Microwave on HIGH 1 minute at a time, for about 3 minutes, until the mixture is thick, stirring after each minute to blend well. Spread the lemon topping over the cooled cookie layer. Let cool.

Dust the top of the cookies with confectioners' sugar. Let cool completely and cut into bars.

Peanut Butter–Chocolate Chip–Oatmeal Bars

brown rice flour
MAKES 15 COOKIES

This cookie was inspired by Annie at my publisher's office. We were looking for a perfect cookie to round out the recipes in the book. We opted for her favorite. It may become your favorite, too! Chocolaty and crumbly!

1/3 cup oil, 65 grams

1/2 cup sugar, 100 grams

1 cup brown rice flour, 125 grams

1/4 cup peanut butter, 65 grams

1/2 cup rolled oats, 50 grams

1 egg

1/4 teaspoon baking soda

1 teaspoon baking powder

1/2 teaspoon salt

1 1/4 teaspoons xanthan gum

1 teaspoon vanilla

1/2 cup semisweet chocolate chips

Preheat the oven to 350°F. Lightly grease an 8-inch square pan.

In medium-size bowl, combine oil and sugar. Beat well to combine. Add flour and beat well. Scrape down sides of the mixing bowl at least once during mixing. Add remaining ingredients, except chips, and beat well. Continue beating until the dough comes together. Mix in the chips. The dough will be crumbly and shiny.

Press the dough into the pan. Bake for approximately 20 minutes, until lightly browned and a toothpick tests clean.

Raspberry-Cream Cheese Brownies

brown rice flour

MAKES 12 BROWNIES

I didn't think a true brownie could be made with a brown rice flour base. Time and experimentation has once again proven that almost anything is possible with almost any gluten-free flour. These brownies are a little cakey, a little gooey, with a swirl of raspberry and cheesecake. Yum!

⅓ cup oil, 65 grams

½ cup sugar, 100 grams

1 cup brown rice flour, 125 grams

⅓ cup unsweetened cocoa powder, 30 grams

2 eggs

¼ teaspoon baking soda

1 teaspoon baking powder

½ teaspoon salt

½ teaspoon xanthan gum

1 teaspoon vanilla extract

Preheat the oven to 350°F. Lightly grease an 8-inch square baking pan.

In a medium-size bowl, combine the oil and sugar. Beat well. Add the brown rice flour and beat well. Scrape down the sides of the mixing bowl at least once during mixing. Add the remaining batter ingredients and beat well. Continue beating until the dough comes together. The dough will be very soft.

Spread the dough evenly in the prepared pan and set aside.

In a separate mixing bowl, beat the cream cheese, egg yolk, confectioners' sugar, and vanilla until well blended. Drop the mixture by the tablespoonful onto the brownie dough, then drop the raspberry jam atop the cream cheese mixture. Use the back of a spoon to swirl it into the brownie dough. Smooth out the top (it will look messy).

(continues on next page)

| Bar Cookies

RASPBERRY-CREAM CHEESE SWIRL:

4 ounces cream cheese

1 egg yolk

1/2 cup confectioners' sugar, 60 grams

1/2 teaspoon vanilla extract

1/3 cup seedless raspberry jam

TOPPING:

3/4 cup semisweet chocolate chips, 120 grams

Bake for about 25 minutes, until the top is dry and a toothpick tests cleanly. While hot, sprinkle the chocolate chips on top of the brownies and cover with foil or a pan. Once melted, spread the chocolate over the brownies. Let cool completely and cut into bars.

Rice Cereal Bars

This is a very well-known favorite cookie bar. Mine is a not-too-big batch and I've used the microwave to speed up making it! (Just one pan from start to finish, too!) I've included an optional chocolate topping.

½ (10½-ounce) bag mini
   marshmallows, 150 grams
   (3¼ cups)

2 tablespoons butter, cut into
  small chunks

4 cups rice cereal

TOPPING (OPTIONAL):
1 cup chocolate chips,
   160 grams

Lightly grease a microwave-safe 8- or 9-inch pan (Pyrex is great). Place the marshmallows and butter in the pan. Microwave on HIGH for 1½ to 2 minutes to melt the marshmallows, stopping after 1 minute to stir. When melted, stir well to fully incorporate the butter. Add the rice cereal and mix in until fully coated. With oiled fingertips, press the mixture flat into the pan.

If desired, melt the chocolate chips in a microwave-safe cup or bowl for about 1½ minutes. (Chocolate chips can retain their shape even though melted; it is important to stir them to see if they are fully melted.) Stir well and spread over the top of the rice cookies. Let cool completely and cut into bars.

Rice Cereal Bars, Peanut Butter

MAKES 16 COOKIES

*I've included a little melted chocolate to drizzle over the top
to make these bars look pretty.*

½ (10½-ounce) bag mini
   marshmallows, 150 grams
   (3¼ cups)
⅓ cup peanut butter
½ teaspoon vanilla extract
3½ cups rice cereal
¼ cup chocolate chips,
   40 grams (optional)

Lightly grease a microwave-safe 8- or 9-inch pan (Pyrex is great). Place the marshmallows, peanut butter, and vanilla in the pan. Microwave on HIGH for 1½ to 2 minutes to melt the marshmallows, stopping after 1 minute to stir. When melted, stir well to fully incorporate the peanut butter. Add the rice cereal and mix in until fully coated. With oiled fingertips, press the mixture flat into the pan.

If desired, melt the chocolate chips in a microwave-safe cup or bowl for 30 to 45 seconds and drizzle on top of the bars. Let cool completely and cut into bars.

Shortbread

brown rice flour
MAKES 12 COOKIES

Great traditional shortbread has so few ingredients: just butter, sugar, flour, and maybe a little salt. It is necessary to use a few extra ingredients to duplicate that incredible cookie, but it is so worth it. This would make an incredible base for a fresh fruit tart, too!

$^1/_3$ cup butter, 70 grams

$^1/_2$ cup sugar, 100 grams

$1^1/_2$ cups brown rice flour, 185 grams

1 egg

2 teaspoons baking powder

$^1/_2$ teaspoon salt

$1^1/_2$ teaspoons xanthan gum

$^1/_2$ teaspoon vanilla extract

Preheat the oven to 350°F. Lightly grease a 9-inch round baking pan or springform pan. In a medium-size bowl, combine the butter and sugar. Beat well. Add the brown rice flour and beat well. Scrape down the sides of the mixing bowl at least once during mixing. Add all the remaining ingredients and mix well. The dough will form lots of small clumps but will not quite come together to form a ball; this is okay. Scrape down the bowl and mix just a little longer to be sure all is mixed well.

Transfer the dough to the prepared pan and press to form a solid, even layer at the bottom of the pan. Prick the dough with a fork.

Bake the shortbread for about 15 minutes, until it has the slightest hint of color at the edge of the pan. Let cool. Cut into pretty wedges before serving.

Toffee Bars

brown rice flour

MAKES 25 COOKIES

Made with a shortbread cookie base, this cookie is topped with toffee and melted chocolate. Delish.

$^{1}/_{3}$ cup butter, 70 grams

$^{1}/_{2}$ cup sugar, 100 grams

1$^{1}/_{2}$ cups brown rice flour, 185 grams

1 egg

2 teaspoons baking powder

$^{1}/_{2}$ teaspoon salt

1$^{1}/_{2}$ teaspoons xanthan gum

$^{1}/_{2}$ teaspoon vanilla extract

TOPPING:

$^{1}/_{2}$ cup brown sugar

$^{1}/_{3}$ cup butter

$^{3}/_{4}$ cup chopped pecans, 120 grams

1 cup chocolate chips, 160 grams

Preheat the oven to 350°F. Lightly grease an 8-inch square baking pan.

In a medium-size bowl, combine the butter and sugar. Beat well. Add the brown rice flour and beat well. Scrape down the sides of the mixing bowl at least once during mixing. Add the remaining batter ingredients and mix well. The dough will form lots of small clumps but will not quite come together to form a ball; this is okay. Scrape down the bowl and mix just a little longer to be sure all is mixed well.

Transfer the dough to the prepared pan and press to form a solid, even layer at the bottom of the pan. Prick the dough with a fork.

Bake the shortbread for about 15 minutes, until it has the slightest hint of color at the edge of the pan. Set aside while preparing the topping.

To make the topping, combine the brown sugar and butter in a small saucepan. Bring to a boil and cook for 7 minutes, stirring constantly. (This mixture becomes exceedingly hot, so be careful that it does not come into contact with your skin! Also, please know that the sugar and butter will blend together, despite not seeming to at first.) Pour this toffee mixture over the cookie base and spread it evenly.

Immediately sprinkle the nuts and chocolate chips over the hot toffee layer. Cover the pan with foil or a baking sheet to allow the chips to melt, then spread them lightly with a knife. Let cool. Cut these into small pieces, as these bars are quite rich.

| Bar Cookies

Trail Mix Bars

This recipe is essentially a rice cereal bar that is chock full of good trail mix ingredients. I think you will like it much more than the cereal bars available in most grocery stores. This recipe uses the standard chocolate, nuts, and raisins, but you can use other dried fruits, nuts, and even coconut to make the recipe your own.

$\frac{1}{2}$ (10$\frac{1}{2}$-ounce) bag mini marshmallows, 150 grams (3$\frac{1}{4}$ cups)

2 tablespoons butter, cut into small chunks

3$\frac{1}{2}$ cups rice cereal

$\frac{3}{4}$ cup raisins, 120 grams

$\frac{3}{4}$ cup M&M's

$\frac{3}{4}$ cup salted peanuts, 85 grams

Lightly grease a microwave-safe 8- or 9-inch pan (Pyrex is great). Place the marshmallows and butter in the pan. Microwave on HIGH for 1$\frac{1}{2}$ to 2 minutes to melt the marshmallows, stopping after 1 minute to stir. When melted, stir well to fully incorporate the butter. Add the rice cereal, raisins, and M&M's. Mix in until fully coated. Stir in the peanuts. With oiled fingertips, press the cookie mixture flat into the pan. Let cool completely and cut into bars.

Turtle Bars

brown rice flour

MAKES 15 COOKIES

A tender cookie layer topped with a chocolate cookie layer full of caramel, chocolate, and nuts, all covered with chocolate.

BASE LAYER:

$^1/_3$ cup shortening, 70 grams

$^1/_2$ cup sugar, 100 grams

$1^1/_2$ cups brown rice flour, 185 grams

1 egg

$^1/_2$ teaspoon salt

$^1/_4$ teaspoon baking soda

2 teaspoons baking powder

1 teaspoon xanthan gum

$^1/_2$ teaspoon vanilla extract

SECOND LAYER:

$^1/_3$ of dough from base layer

1 tablespoon unsweetened cocoa powder

2 tablespoons oil

1 egg yolk

5 soft caramel candies, chopped, 40 grams

$^1/_4$ cup chopped chocolate chips, 40 grams

$^1/_4$ cup chopped peanuts (optional), 40 grams

TOPPING:

$^1/_2$ cup chocolate chips, 80 grams

Preheat the oven to 350°F. Lightly grease an 8-inch square baking pan.

In a medium-size bowl, combine the shortening and sugar. Beat well. Add the brown rice flour and beat well. Scrape down the sides of the mixing bowl at least once during mixing. Add the remaining base layer ingredients and mix well, until the dough comes together. Press two-thirds of the dough (about 260 grams) evenly into the prepared pan. Set aside.

For the second layer, combine the retained third of dough with the cocoa, oil, and egg yolk. Mix well. Mix in the caramel, chocolate pieces, and nuts (if desired).

Bake for about 25 minutes. After removing from the oven, sprinkle the bars with the chocolate chips and cover the pan with foil to melt the chips. Once soft, spread the chocolate over the bars. Let cool completely and cut into bars.

White Chocolate Bars

brown rice flour

MAKES 20 COOKIES

A tender cookie layer topped with a white chocolate fudgelike topping. For extra flavor, add a layer of chopped raisins or macadamia nuts before applying the white chocolate top layer. These are very rich cookie bars.

⅓ cup butter, 70 grams

½ cup sugar, 100 grams

1½ cups brown rice flour, 185 grams

1 egg

2 teaspoons baking powder

½ teaspoon salt

1½ teaspoons xanthan gum

1 teaspoon vanilla extract

OPTIONAL MIDDLE LAYER:
½ cup chopped raisins (optional), 80 grams

½ cup chopped macadamia nuts (optional), 65 grams

Preheat the oven to 350°F. Lightly grease an 8-inch square baking pan.

In a medium-size bowl, combine the butter and sugar. Beat well. Add the brown rice flour and beat well. Scrape down the sides of the mixing bowl at least once during mixing. Add the remaining base layer ingredients and mix well. The dough will form lots of small clumps but will not quite come together to form a ball; this is okay. Scrape down the bowl and mix just a little longer to be sure all is mixed well.

Transfer the dough to the prepared pan and press to form a solid, even layer at the bottom of the pan. Add the layer of chopped raisins and/or nuts, if desired.

TOPPING:
1$\frac{1}{2}$ tablespoons cherry juice
1 cup white chocolate chips
$\frac{1}{2}$ cup sweetened condensed milk

In a microwave-safe cup, combine the cherry juice, white chocolate chips, and condensed milk. Microwave on HIGH for 1$\frac{1}{2}$ to 2 minutes, stirring frequently, until the chocolate melts and is of spreading consistency. Pour the mixture over the cookie layers, tilting the pan to reach the edges.

Bake for about 18 minutes, until the edges begin to lightly brown. Let cool completely and cut into bars.

5

Rolled and Piped Cookies

Beautiful cookies! This chapter is full of beautiful cookies! The Butter Cookies and Chocolate Butter Cookies are easy to pipe spritz-style cookies—classics. And for smiles that only S'mores can bring, there are Graham Crackers, traditional and chocolate! One of the prettiest cookies of all is the Linzer Sandwich Cookie with jam peeking out of a window dusted with confectioners' sugar.

The most important thing to remember when working with these special cookies is patience, whether you are placing the cookie dough in the fridge for easier handling, or rolling and cutting out shapes.

I have found it easiest to roll out cookies on a lightly oiled surface, using a lightly oiled rolling pin. I use nonstick spray to coat the surfaces. And, although it is certainly not necessary, granite is my surface of choice. It stays naturally cool to the touch. An 18-inch square of granite tile or smooth ceramic tile can be acquired from your local hardware store at minimal cost.

Animal Crackers

brown rice flour and cornstarch

MAKES ABOUT 150 COOKIES

I think I've eaten one too many cookies! I was testing the "real" Barnum's Animal Crackers and noticed an underlying corn taste. I hadn't noticed that in all my years of eating these treats, so I checked the label. Yes, yellow corn flour is one of the ingredients. We'll use a little cornstarch since we already have the grit from brown rice flour. These cookies are a little more tender than the original, but are delicious—not to mention fun to make. Finding tiny cookie cutters might be the hardest thing about making these cookies!

¹/₃ cup oil, 65 grams

¹/₂ cup light brown sugar, 100 grams

1 cup brown rice flour, 125 grams

¹/₃ cup cornstarch, 40 grams

2 egg yolks

¹/₄ teaspoon baking soda

¹/₂ teaspoon salt

1 teaspoon xanthan gum

1 teaspoon vanilla extract

1¹/₂ tablespoons water

Preheat the oven to 350°F. Lightly grease a cookie sheet.

In a medium-size bowl, combine the oil and sugar. Beat well. Add the brown rice flour and cornstarch and beat well. Scrape down the sides of the mixing bowl at least once during mixing. Add the remaining ingredients and beat well. Continue beating until the dough comes together; it will be soft and oily to the touch.

Roll out the dough to ¹/₈-inch thickness. Use tiny 1-inch cookie cutters to cut the cookies. The dough is very easy to work with, but quite soft. Place the cookies on the prepared pan.

Bake the animal crackers for 10 to 12 minutes, until the tops are lightly browned. Avoid both overbaking and underbaking. Let cool on wire racks before serving.

Butter Cookies

brown rice flour
MAKES ABOUT 60 COOKIES

Very buttery, delicate, not-too-sweet cookies.
I use a cookie press to make these pretty cookies.

½ cup butter, 110 grams

½ cup sugar, 100 grams

1½ cups brown rice flour, 185 grams

1 egg, plus 1 egg yolk

¼ teaspoon baking soda

1 teaspoon baking powder

½ teaspoon salt

1 teaspoon xanthan gum

1 teaspoon vanilla extract

Preheat the oven to 350°F. Very lightly grease a cookie sheet. (Overgreasing will prevent the cookie dough from adhering during pressing. Wipe off extra oil if necessary.)

In a medium-size bowl, combine the butter and sugar. Beat well. Add the brown rice flour and beat well. Scrape down the sides of the mixing bowl at least once during mixing. Add the remaining ingredients and beat well. Continue beating until the dough comes together; it will be soft and almost creamy.

Place the dough in a cookie press and "shoot" the cookies onto the prepared pan. Alternatively, the dough may be piped from a pastry bag.

Bake the cookies for about 10 minutes, until the edges begin to brown. Let cool on wire racks before serving.

Candy Cane Cookies

brown rice flour

MAKES ABOUT 25 COOKIES

These cookies are cut from strips of colored dough that are rolled flat into a striped mat, making for a prettier cookie than twisting strips of dough together. As with the Chinese Marble Cookies, this recipe avoids using butter. By using oil (shortening in the case of the Chinese Marble Cookies) the clean essence of other flavors shine.

⅓ cup oil, 65 grams

½ cup plus 2 tablespoons sugar, 125 grams

1½ cups brown rice flour, 185 grams

1 egg

¼ teaspoon baking soda

1 teaspoon baking powder

½ teaspoon salt

1 teaspoon xanthan gum

3 tablespoons water

½ teaspoon vanilla extract

½ teaspoon peppermint extract

About ¼ teaspoon red paste food coloring

TOPPING:
1 tablespoon sugar

Preheat the oven to 350°F. Lightly grease a cookie sheet.

In a medium-size bowl, combine the oil and sugar. Beat well. Add the brown rice flour and beat well. Scrape down the sides of the mixing bowl at least once during mixing. Add the remaining ingredients and beat well. Continue beating until the dough comes together.

Divide the dough in half. Set half of the dough (about 250 grams) aside. Mix a little red food coloring into the remaining half of the dough until the desired color is reached. Refrigerate both batches of dough for at least 30 minutes, for easier handling.

Roll each section of the dough flat, about ¼-
inch thick. Cut the dough into thin strips
and then lay down alternating colored strips
side by side to form a tight, striped dough
mat. Roll it slightly to be sure that the dough
strips seal to each other. Finally, cut the
dough at a 45-degree angle to form thin strips
with a slanted angle of stripes showing. Cut
the strips into 5-inch lengths and place them
on the prepared pan. Gently bend the top of
each 5-inch length sideways to form the arch
of the candy cane. Sprinkle the tops lightly
with plain sugar.

Bake the cookies for about 10 minutes, until the
tops just begin to take on a little color. Let
cool on wire racks before serving.

Chinese Marble Cookies

brown rice flour

MAKES ABOUT 18 COOKIES

I was introduced to Chinese Marble Cookies at a beautiful dance pavilion in Maryland, thanks to Steve, a great dance instructor. These cookies have chocolate "marbling" throughout a very light-colored cookie base. These cookies taste like a cross between a sugar cookie and shortbread, with dark chocolate thrown in for good measure. The character of the cookie changes entirely if butter is substituted, so stick with shortening. I love butter, but not in these cookies.

¹/₃ cup shortening, 70 grams

¹/₂ cup sugar, 100 grams

1¹/₂ cups brown rice flour, 185 grams

1 egg

2 teaspoons baking powder

¹/₂ teaspoon salt

1 teaspoon xanthan gum

¹/₂ teaspoon vanilla extract

1¹/₂ teaspoons water

1 square (1 ounce) unsweetened chocolate

Preheat the oven to 350°F. Lightly grease a cookie sheet.

In a medium-size bowl, combine the shortening and sugar. Beat well. Add the brown rice flour and beat well. Scrape down the sides of the mixing bowl at least once during mixing. Add the remaining ingredients, except for the chocolate, and mix well. The cookie dough will form large clumps, but will not quite come together to form a ball; this is okay.

Melt the chocolate in a microwave-safe bowl or cup in a microwave on HIGH for about 1 minute. Pour it over the dough and stir it in with a few swirls of a fork just until a marbled effect occurs (do not overmix).

Roll out the dough to ¼-inch thickness and cut it with a 2½-inch round cookie cutter (or other cookie cutter of your choice).

Bake the cookies for 9 to 10 minutes, until they have the slightest hint of color. The tops will be dry. Let cool on wire racks before serving.

Chocolate Butter Cookies

brown rice flour

MAKES ABOUT 50 COOKIES

It is almost unbelievable that such a cookie can be made using brown rice flour as the base. Gluten-free just gets better and better! Choose your favorite chocolate to drizzle over the top. This cookie flavor is best at room temperature; it is more buttery when warm.

1/2 cup butter, 110 grams

1/2 cup sugar, 100 grams

1 1/4 cups brown rice flour, 155 grams

1/4 cup unsweetened cocoa powder, 20 grams

1 egg, plus 1 egg yolk

1/4 teaspoon baking soda

1/2 teaspoon salt

1 teaspoon xanthan gum

1 teaspoon vanilla extract

1 tablespoon water

TOPPING (OPTIONAL):
2 ounces chocolate

Preheat the oven to 350°F. Very lightly grease a cookie sheet.

In a medium-size bowl, combine the butter and sugar. Beat well. Add the brown rice flour and beat well. Scrape down the sides of the mixing bowl at least once during mixing. Add the remaining ingredients and beat well. Continue beating until the dough comes together; it will be soft and almost creamy.

Place the dough in a pastry bag and pipe the cookies onto the prepared pan. Bake for about 12 minutes, until the edges begin to brown and the cookies lose their sheen. Let cool on wire racks.

For the topping, break up the chocolate into a microwave-safe cup or bowl. Melt, stirring often, in the microwave on HIGH for up to 1 minute. As the container may be very hot, use care as you dip the tines of a fork into the melted chocolate and drizzle it over the cookies.

Chocolate Graham Crackers

brown rice flour

MAKES 10 TO 12 LARGE GRAHAM CRACKERS

It's funny to use the word graham in the name of this cookie as graham flour is wheat flour, but no matter, it is the very description you need to visualize this cookie style. This wheat-free graham cracker is richly chocolaty and not too sweet.

1/3 cup shortening, 70 grams

1 cup brown rice flour, 125 grams

1/2 cup brown sugar, 100 grams

1/3 cup cocoa, 30 grams

1 egg white

Scant 1/2 teaspoon baking soda

1/2 teaspoon salt

1 teaspoon xanthan gum

1/4 teaspoon vanilla extract

Preheat the oven to 350°F. Lightly grease a cookie sheet.

In a medium-size bowl, combine the shortening and brown rice flour. Beat well. Scrape down the sides of the mixing bowl at least once during mixing. Add the remaining ingredients and beat well. Continue beating until the dough is thick and heavy. Continue beating for an additional 30 seconds to 1 minute for additional dough stability.

Roll out the dough to 1/8-inch thickness. Using a pizza cutter, cut the dough into 5 by 2¼-inch rectangles and place them on the prepared pan. Lightly score each cracker with a lengthwise and a crosswise indentation (to quarter each cracker), not cutting all the way through. Prick the tops of the crackers with a fork.

(continues on next page)

Bake for about 9 minutes. As the crackers crisp during cooling and it is hard to tell what browning is taking place under that cocoa color, the proof is in the cooled cracker. I suggest you bake one as a test to determine the exact, best baking time—not enough leaves a slightly soft (although delicious) cookie; too much leaves an overly crisp cracker. Let cool on wire racks before serving.

Chocolate Meringues

Most meringue recipes call for cream of tartar to stabilize the meringue structure. In this recipe, we are able to omit it. These cookies are light and airy on the outside and almost a little fudgy on the inside. A fat-free winner!

2 egg whites, 65 grams
(at room temperature)

$1/3$ cup sugar, 75 grams

$1/2$ teaspoon vanilla extract

$1/4$ cup unsweetened cocoa
powder, 20 grams

Preheat the oven to 300°F. Lightly grease a cookie sheet.

In a medium-size bowl, beat the egg whites, sugar, and vanilla until the whites form stiff peaks (This takes several minutes, depending upon the strength of your mixer. It also takes longer for stiff peaks to form with the inclusion of the sugar than if the egg whites were beaten alone.) The batter will look like marshmallow cream. Sprinkle the cocoa on the batter and gently fold it in. The dough will then look like whipped cream.

Using a piping bag with a large star tip, pipe large stars of dough onto the prepared pan, or just drop rounded teaspoonfuls of dough onto the pan. Bake the cookies for 15 to 20 minutes, until the bottom edges just begin to brown (which is hard to tell on this chocolate version) and the tops appear dry. Let cool on wire racks before serving.

Chocolate Pinwheel Cookies

brown rice flour

MAKES ABOUT 25 COOKIES

A spiral of two tender cookies that complement each other well. What could be better than both chocolate and vanilla in a not-too-sweet cookie?

½ cup butter, 110 grams

½ cup sugar, 100 grams

1¼ cups brown rice flour, 155 grams, plus 2 tablespoons, 15 grams

1 egg, plus 1 egg yolk

¼ teaspoon baking soda

½ teaspoon salt

1 teaspoon xanthan gum

1 teaspoon vanilla extract

½ teaspoon baking powder

2 tablespoons unsweetened cocoa powder, 10 grams

Preheat the oven to 350°F. Lightly grease a cookie sheet.

In a medium-size bowl, combine the butter and sugar. Beat well. Add the 1¼ cups of brown rice flour and beat well. Scrape down the sides of the mixing bowl at least once during mixing. Add the egg, egg yolk, baking soda, salt, xanthan gum, and vanilla, and beat well. Continue beating until the dough comes together; it will be soft and almost creamy.

Remove half of the dough (220 grams) from the mixing bowl and set it aside in another bowl. To the dough remaining in the bowl, add the remaining 2 tablespoons of brown rice flour and the baking powder and mix well. Set aside. To the other half of the dough, add the cocoa and mix well. Set aside. Both batches of dough may be refrigerated for 30 minutes for easier handling.

Pat the lighter dough on a lightly greased surface (waxed paper is nice) to form a 12 by 6-inch rectangle. Top the lighter dough with the darker dough, creating one rectangle with two layers. Roll the dough into a long log, rolling from the longer side, to create a spiral effect. Refrigerate the log until firm, about 30 minutes.

Slice the dough into ⅓- to ½-inch slices and place them on the prepared pan.

Bake the pinwheels for 10 to 12 minutes, until the edges begin to brown. Let cool on wire racks before serving.

Chocolate Wafer Hearts

sorghum flour

MAKES ABOUT 24 COOKIES

Tender, very chocolaty cookies. Imagine a chocolate version of a rolled sugar cookie . . . yep, that good. Drizzle with a little melted chocolate if desired. If you are avoiding rice flour, these make an ideal substitute for the base cookie used in Oreos-Style Cookies (page 116).

⅓ cup oil, 65 grams

½ cup sugar, 100 grams

1 cup sorghum flour, 135 grams

⅓ cup unsweetened cocoa powder, 30 grams

1 egg

¼ teaspoon baking soda

½ teaspoon salt

½ teaspoon xanthan gum

1 teaspoon vanilla extract

Preheat the oven to 350°F. Lightly grease a cookie sheet.

In a medium-size bowl, combine the oil and sugar. Beat well. Add the sorghum flour and cocoa and beat well. Scrape down the sides of the mixing bowl at least once during mixing. Add the remaining ingredients and mix well. Continue beating until the dough comes together. The dough will be oily, yet seem almost too dry.

Roll out the dough to no more than ¼-inch thickness. Cut it with a 2¼-inch heart-shaped cookie cutter or other favorite cookie cutter.

Bake for 8 minutes, until the cookies lose their sheen. Let cool on wire racks before serving.

Cinnabon-Style Cookies

brown rice flour

MAKES ABOUT 24 COOKIES

Inspired by those famous buns at the mall, these cookies are buttery, tender, and full of cinnamon flavor.

⅓ cup shortening, 70 grams

½ cup sugar, 100 grams

1½ cups brown rice flour, 185 grams

1 egg

¼ teaspoon baking soda

2 teaspoons baking powder

½ teaspoon salt

1 teaspoon xanthan gum

1 teaspoon vanilla extract

1½ teaspoons water

CINNAMON-SUGAR MIXTURE:

2 tablespoons butter, very soft

1 teaspoon ground cinnamon

2 tablespoons brown sugar

GLAZE:

⅔ cup confectioners' sugar

1 tablespoon water

Preheat the oven to 350°F. Lightly grease a cookie sheet.

In a medium-size bowl, combine the shortening and sugar. Beat well. Add the brown rice flour and beat well. Scrape down the sides of the mixing bowl at least once during mixing. Add the remaining batter ingredients. The cookie dough will form large clumps, but will not quite come together to form a ball; this is okay.

On a sheet of waxed paper, roll out the dough to a ¼-inch-thick, 8 by 11-inch rectangle. Spread the butter, then the cinnamon and sugar over the rolled dough. Roll up the dough into a snug, long tube, rolling from the longer side, and slice it into ¼-inch rounds. Place them on the prepared pan.

Bake the cookies for 11 to 13 minutes, until the tops are lightly browned. Let cool on wire racks.

Combine the glaze ingredients in a small cup and stir well. Drizzle the glaze over the tops of the cookies.

Crisp Almond Cookies

brown rice flour and almond meal

MAKES ABOUT 25 COOKIES

These crisp cookies have the wonderful flavor of almonds complemented by a substantial partial dipping in dark chocolate. These cookies are delicious even without the extra chocolate.

$1/3$ cup shortening, 70 grams

$1/2$ cup sugar, 100 grams

1 cup brown rice flour, 125 grams

1 egg, plus 1 egg yolk

$1/2$ cup almond meal, 60 grams

$1/4$ teaspoon baking soda

2 teaspoons baking powder

$1/2$ teaspoon salt

1 teaspoon xanthan gum

1 teaspoon almond extract

TOPPING (OPTIONAL):

4 to 6 ounces dark chocolate, melted

$1/4$ cup sliced almonds

Preheat the oven to 350°F. Lightly grease a cookie sheet.

In a medium-size bowl, combine the shortening and sugar. Beat well. Add the brown rice flour and beat well. Scrape down the sides of the mixing bowl at least once during mixing. Add the remaining batter ingredients and mix well. The dough will be quite thick.

Roll the dough to $1/8$- to $1/4$-inch thickness and cut it with a 2-inch round cookie cutter (or other cookie cutter of your choice).

Bake the cookies for 8 to 10 minutes, until they have the slightest hint of color; the tops will be dry. Let cool on wire racks.

In a microwave-safe dish, melt 2 ounces of chocolate at a time. Dip or brush half of each cookie with chocolate and place on waxed paper to firm up. Sprinkle with a few sliced almonds, if desired.

Gingerbread Men and Gingersnaps

brown rice flour and sorghum flour

MAKES ABOUT 16 SMALL GINGERBREAD MEN OR 32 GINGERSNAPS

As gingerbread men, these cookies are sturdy, crisp, not-too-sweet, and quite tasty. I use a hint of vanilla to soften the bitterness of the ground ginger. As gingersnaps, these cookies have a light sprinkling of sugar and definitely have a snap to their texture.

$\frac{1}{3}$ cup shortening, 70 grams

$\frac{1}{2}$ cup sugar, 100 grams

2 tablespoons unsulfured molasses

$\frac{3}{4}$ cup brown rice flour, 95 grams

$\frac{3}{4}$ cup sorghum flour, 100 grams

$\frac{1}{2}$ teaspoon baking soda

$\frac{1}{2}$ teaspoon salt

1 teaspoon xanthan gum

$\frac{3}{4}$ teaspoon ground ginger

$\frac{1}{2}$ teaspoon vanilla extract (optional)

1 egg

TOPPING FOR GINGERBREAD MEN:
Icing and/or candies

TOPPING FOR GINGERSNAPS:
2 tablespoons sugar

Preheat the oven to 375°F. Lightly grease a cookie sheet.

In a medium-size bowl, combine the shortening, sugar, and molasses. Beat well. Scrape down the sides of the mixing bowl at least once during mixing. Add the remaining batter ingredients and beat well. The batter will form a soft dough; continue to beat it for about 30 seconds after it forms, to stabilize the dough.

For gingerbread men, roll out the dough on a lightly greased surface to $\frac{1}{8}$-inch thickness. Cut with a cookie cutter and place the cookies on the prepared pan.

For gingersnaps, drop rounded teaspoonfuls of the dough on the prepared pan and press to just under $\frac{1}{4}$-inch thickness. Sprinkle lightly with sugar.

Bake the cookies for 7 to 8 minutes, until the edges are lightly browned.

The cookies will crisp during cooling. Let cool on wire racks. Decorate with icing and candies as desired.

Graham Crackers

brown rice flour

MAKES 10 TO 12 LARGE GRAHAM CRACKERS

These classic crackers are tender, crisp, and easy to make.
S'mores are back on the bonfire menu! Top them with a little cinnamon sugar
for another tasty alternative.

¹/₃ cup shortening, 70 grams

1¹/₂ cups brown rice flour,
   185 grams

¹/₂ cup brown sugar, 100 grams

1 egg white

¹/₂ teaspoon baking soda

¹/₂ teaspoon salt

1 teaspoon xanthan gum

Preheat the oven to 350°F. Lightly grease a cookie sheet.

In a medium-size bowl, combine the shortening and brown rice flour. Beat well. Scrape down the sides of the mixing bowl at least once during mixing. Add the remaining ingredients and beat well. Continue beating until the dough is thick and heavy. It should not fall apart easily.

Roll out the dough to ¹/₈-inch thickness. Using a pizza cutter, cut it into large 5 by 2¹/₄-inch rectangles and place them on the prepared pan. Lightly score each cracker with a lengthwise and a crosswise indentation (to quarter each cracker), not cutting all the way through. Prick the tops of the crackers with a fork.

Bake the graham crackers for 8 to 10 minutes, until the edges are lightly browned and the tops just begin to brown. The crackers will crisp during cooling. Underbaking leaves the cooled cracker slightly soft and overbaking makes it just a little too crisp. My test crackers were perfect at 9 minutes. Let cool on wire racks before serving.

Note: Should you have difficulty in handling the dough, you can roll it out directly on the baking sheet, then cut the rectangles and remove the excess dough. I like to make other shapes as well: circles, hearts, whatever. Please note that the more you handle this dough, the easier it becomes to work with . . . with no ill effects on the cookie. (You can't say that about a traditional cookie!)

| Rolled and Piped Cookies

Ice-Cream Sandwich Cookies

brown rice flour

MAKES ABOUT 11 SANDWICH COOKIES

Not quite cakelike, not quite cookielike. For simplicity, I make these cookies round. Tasty alone, they're even better with a scoop of ice cream sandwiched between two cookies just before serving.

1/3 cup oil, 65 grams

3/4 cup sugar, 150 grams

1 cup brown rice flour, 125 grams

1/3 cup unsweetened cocoa powder, 30 grams

1 egg

1/4 cup plain yogurt, 60 grams

1/4 teaspoon baking soda

1/2 teaspoon salt

1 teaspoon xanthan gum

1 teaspoon vanilla extract

Preheat the oven to 350°F. Lightly grease a cookie sheet.

In a medium-size bowl, combine the oil and sugar. Beat well. Add the brown rice flour and beat well. Add the remaining ingredients and mix well. The dough will be very thick, but still thin enough for rolling out.

Drop tablespoonfuls of dough onto the prepared pan. Using moistened fingertips, press it to 1/8-inch thickness. Prick the tops of the cookies with a fork. Or, for a prettier presentation, press the tops with a fondant cutter.

Bake for 10 minutes, until the cookies take on a bit of color at the edges and the tops appear dry. Let cool. The cookies will be very soft when removing them from the baking sheet, but will firm during cooling. Let cool on wire racks before serving.

Lady Fingers

brown rice flour

MAKES ABOUT 30 COOKIES

Light and airy, I would call them even a little poofy. Sandwich two of these together with the lemon curd created as part of the Lemon Tassies recipe on page 130. Awesome.

$^{1}/_{3}$ cup oil, 65 grams

$^{1}/_{2}$ cup sugar, 10 grams

1 cup brown rice flour, 125 grams

$^{1}/_{2}$ cup plain yogurt, 120 grams

1 teaspoon baking soda

$^{1}/_{2}$ teaspoon salt

$^{3}/_{4}$ teaspoon xanthan gum

1 teaspoon vanilla extract

1 egg yolk

2 egg whites

TOPPING:
2 tablespoons confectioners' sugar

Preheat the oven to 350°F. Lightly grease a cookie sheet.

In a medium-size bowl, combine the oil and sugar. Beat well. Add the brown rice flour and beat well. Scrape down the sides of the mixing bowl at least once during mixing. Add the remaining batter ingredients, except the egg whites, and mix well. The dough will be like a thick cake batter. Set aside.

Separately, beat the egg whites until stiff peaks form. (This will take several minutes, depending upon the temperature of the egg whites and the strength of the mixer.) Gently fold them into the batter.

Transfer the batter into a zip-type plastic bag. Cut off a $^{1}/_{2}$-inch angle at one corner. Pipe 3- to $3^{1}/_{2}$-inch long fingers onto the prepared pan.

Bake for 8 to 10 minutes, until browned at edges and the sponge is firm. Let cool briefly on the pan for easier removal and then cool on wire racks before serving.

Lemon Meringues

Inspired by lemon meringue pie, I just couldn't resist trying this out! To make these cookies extra special, make the lemon curd that is part of the Lemon Tassies recipe on page 130, and sandwich a bit of it between two lemon meringues. They taste like a lemon cloud.

2 egg whites, 65 grams

1/3 cup sugar, 75 grams

1 teaspoon lemon extract

Preheat the oven to 300°F. Lightly grease a cookie sheet.

In a medium-size bowl, beat the egg whites and sugar until the whites form stiff peaks. (This will take several minutes, depending upon the temperature of the egg whites and the strength of the mixer. It takes longer for stiff peaks to form with the inclusion of the sugar than if egg whites were beaten alone.) The batter will look like marshmallow cream. Beat in the lemon extract. Do not underbeat, as the shape of cookie relies upon the ability of the meringue to hold its shape!

Using a piping bag with a large star tip, pipe a small star onto the prepared pan, or just drop rounded teaspoonfuls of the dough onto the pan. Bake the cookies for 15 to 20 minutes, until the bottom edges just begin to brown and the tops look dry. Let cool on wire racks before serving.

Linzer Sandwich Cookies

brown rice flour and almond meal

MAKES ABOUT 17 SANDWICH COOKIES

Your favorite jam sandwiched between two crisp nut cookies, dusted with a little confectioners' sugar. Be sure to cut a small "window" in half of the cookies so the jam peeks out. Very pretty! These cookies lose some crispness once filled, so fill these shortly before serving if possible.

$\frac{1}{3}$ cup shortening, 70 grams

$\frac{1}{2}$ cup sugar, 100 grams

1 cup brown rice flour, 125 grams

1 egg

$\frac{1}{2}$ cup almond meal, 60 grams

$\frac{1}{2}$ teaspoon baking powder

$\frac{1}{2}$ teaspoon salt

1$\frac{1}{2}$ teaspoons xanthan gum

$\frac{1}{2}$ teaspoon almond extract

TOPPING:

$\frac{1}{2}$ cup seedless raspberry jam, or other favorite jam

$\frac{1}{4}$ cup confectioners' sugar

Preheat the oven to 350°F. Lightly grease a cookie sheet.

In a medium-size bowl, combine the shortening and sugar. Beat well. Add the brown rice flour and beat well. Scrape down the sides of the mixing bowl at least once during mixing. Add the remaining ingredients and mix well. The dough will form lots of small clumps, and, with continued beating, will come together.

Roll out the dough to $\frac{1}{8}$-inch thickness and cut it into 2-inch circles. Using a smaller cookie cutter, cut a small window in the center of half of the cookies. Place the cookies on the prepared pan.

Bake the cookies for about 8 minutes, until the edges begin to lightly brown. Let cool on wire racks. Place a small amount of jam on the bottoms of the full-circle cookies. Sprinkle the cookie tops (the ones with windows) with confectioners' sugar. Gently sandwich in pairs to form sugar-topped, jam-filled cookies.

Nut Meringue Wreaths

almond meal

MAKES 20 TO 30 COOKIES

I've used almond meal for this recipe as it is readily available. Although these meringues may be piped or spooned into any shape, wreaths make a pretty presentation for the holiday season.

2 egg whites, 65 grams

1/3 cup sugar, 75 grams

1/4 teaspoon cream of tartar

1/2 teaspoon vanilla extract

1/4 cup almond meal, 30 grams

TOPPING (OPTIONAL):
Almond slices or bits

Preheat the oven to 300°F. Lightly grease a cookie sheet.

In a medium-size bowl, beat the egg whites, about half of the sugar, the cream of tartar, and vanilla, until the whites form stiff peaks. (This will take several minutes, depending upon the temperature of the egg whites and the strength of the mixer. It takes longer for stiff peaks to form with the inclusion of the sugar than if egg whites were beaten alone.) The batter will look like marshmallow cream. Sprinkle the almond meal and remaining sugar on the batter and gently fold them in. The dough will now look like whipped cream.

Using a piping bag with a circle tip (or a zip-type plastic bag with a corner cut off), pipe wreath-shaped cookies onto the prepared pan and garnish with almond slices or bits. Bake for 15 to 20 minutes, until the bottom edges just begin to brown and the tops look dry. Let cool on wire racks before serving.

Rolled Sugar Cookies

brown rice flour

MAKES ABOUT 30 TWO-INCH COOKIES

These are traditional buttery sugar cookies. You may use all butter, if desired (instead of shortening). When planning to make this recipe, keep in mind that the dough needs to be refrigerated for an hour and you must work very quickly with small portions of dough to achieve sharp cutouts.

1/4 cup butter, 55 grams

1/4 cup shortening, 50 grams

1/2 cup sugar, 100 grams

1 1/2 cups brown rice flour, 185 grams

1 egg, plus 1 egg yolk

1/4 teaspoon baking soda

1/2 teaspoon salt

1 1/4 teaspoons xanthan gum

1 teaspoon vanilla extract

TOPPING:
Sprinkles or colored sugar

Icing (optional)

Preheat the oven to 350°F. Very lightly grease a cookie sheet.

In a medium-size bowl, combine the butter, shortening, and sugar. Beat well. Add the brown rice flour and beat well. Scrape down the sides of the mixing bowl at least once during mixing. Add the remaining ingredients and beat well. Continue beating until the dough comes together. At this stage the dough will be too soft to roll. Refrigerate for 1 hour.

Roll out the dough to between 1/8- and 1/4-inch thickness. Cut it using cookie cutters of your choice and place the cut cookies on the prepared pan. Decorate with sprinkles or colored sugar as desired (or leave bare, if you are planning to ice them later).

Bake the cookies for about 10 minutes, until the edges begin to brown. Let cool on wire racks.

Ice and decorate, if desired.

Rolled Sugar Cookies, Dairy-Free

brown rice flour

MAKES ABOUT 30 COOKIES

Here is a dairy-free version of a rolled sugar cookie.
They are simply delicious.

$^1/_3$ cup shortening, 70 grams

$^1/_2$ cup sugar, 100 grams

$1^1/_2$ cups brown rice flour,
   185 grams

1 egg

$1^1/_2$ teaspoons baking powder

$^1/_2$ teaspoon salt

1 teaspoon xanthan gum

1 teaspoon vanilla extract

$1^1/_2$ teaspoons water

TOPPING (OPTIONAL):
Sprinkles or colored sugar

Preheat the oven to 350°F. Lightly grease a cookie sheet.

In a medium-size bowl, combine the shortening and sugar. Beat well. Add the flour and beat well. Scrape down the sides of the mixing bowl at least once during mixing. Add the remaining ingredients and mix well. The cookie dough will form large clumps, but will not quite come together to form a ball. Press it together with your hands.

Roll out the dough to $^1/_8$- to $^1/_4$-inch thickness and cut it with a 2-inch round cookie cutter (or other cookie cutter of your choice). Place the cookies on the prepared pan. Top with sprinkles or colored sugar, if desired.

Bake the cookies for 8 to 10 minutes, until they have the slightest hint of color and the tops are dry. Let cool on wire racks.

Stained-Glass Cookies

brown rice flour

MAKES ABOUT 25 COOKIES

Use your favorite clear candy (such as lollipops or individual hard candies) for the "glass" in these pretty cookies. Use multiple colors or just one. And expect a casualty or two when removing the cookies from the baking sheet.

1/3 cup oil, 65 grams

1/2 cup sugar, 100 grams

1 1/2 cups brown rice flour, 185 grams

1 egg, plus 1 egg yolk

1/4 teaspoon baking soda

1/2 teaspoon salt

1 teaspoon xanthan gum

1 teaspoon vanilla extract

STAINED GLASS:
About 8 crushed, clear candies

TOPPING (OPTIONAL):
Confectioners' sugar

Preheat the oven to 350°F. Lightly grease a cookie sheet.

In a medium-size bowl, combine the oil and sugar. Beat well. Add the brown rice flour and beat well. Scrape down the sides of the mixing bowl at least once during mixing. Add the remaining batter ingredients and beat well. Continue beating until the dough almost comes together. Press it together with your hands to form a ball. The dough will feel oily.

Roll out the dough flat, to less than 1/4-inch thick. Cut the dough with a 2 1/2-inch cookie cutter and then cut the center of each cookie with another cutter of the same shape, but smaller, to form the window, and remove the center scrap of dough. Place the large cutouts well apart on the prepared pan. The cookies will spread during baking. Fill the windows with a small amount of crushed candy. Reroll the scraps into additional cookies.

(continues on next page)

Bake for 9 to10 minutes, until the cookies begin to take on color. Let cool on the baking sheet to allow the window candy to harden. Sprinkle the tops with confectioners' sugar, if desired.

Note: To crush the candies, place them in a small plastic bag and hit them with a rolling pin or the dull end of a butter knife. Take care while eating these; the candy windowpanes can be sharp when bitten or broken.

6

Great Fakes Cookies

When I first started working on recipes for this book, I wanted to be sure to meet our everyday cravings. Although everyone loves a homemade classic, sometimes a supermarket cookie or Girl Scout cookie is really what is desired! I re-created several of my favorite Girl Scout cookies during "cookie season," but time and time again, I was asked to add just one more.

The Girl Scouts of Central Maryland, Inc., came to my rescue! They provided me with sample packages of cookies so that I could compare my work side-by-side with their delicious varieties. I cannot help but smile that the Girl Scouts gave cookies to help those who will never be able to eat theirs. And, while of course the recipes included in this chapter are not identical to Girl Scout cookies, they are some awesome great fakes!

My local grocery store's cookie aisle (and Trader Joe's) held the rest of the inspiration for this chapter: Oreos, Chips Ahoy!, Nutter Butters, Fig Newtons, and Little Debbie Oatmeal Creme Pies, to name a few. Diverse and delicious in their own way, I have also re-created these beloved favorites.

In making each cookie, I deconstructed the original. Many cookies are not what you think. Sometimes it is just the filling that has the flavor. Other times, you think you are eating a sweet-base cookie only to find it is rather plain and not sweet at all. And oh, the nuances of cream filling! These substitutes are perhaps the greatest proof that almost anything is possible in a gluten-free cookie.

Chips Ahoy!-Style Cookies

brown rice flour

MAKES ABOUT 25 COOKIES

Wandering down the cookie aisle at the grocery store, I thought a lot about which cookies to duplicate. These original, crunchy ones were the first in my cart. I've made these slice-and-bake for the no-fuss kitchen.

¹/₃ cup shortening, 70 grams

¹/₂ cup light brown sugar, 100 grams

1¹/₂ cups brown rice flour, 185 grams

1 egg

¹/₂ teaspoon baking soda

¹/₂ teaspoon salt

1 teaspoon xanthan gum

¹/₂ teaspoon vanilla extract

1 tablespoon water

¹/₂ cup semisweet chocolate morsels, chopped, 80 grams

Preheat the oven to 350°F. Lightly grease a cookie sheet.

In a medium-size bowl, combine the shortening and sugar. Beat well. Add the brown rice flour and mix well. Add the remaining ingredients, except for the chocolate chips, and mix well. The cookie dough will form large clumps, but will not quite come together to form a ball; this is okay. Add the chocolate chips and mix well.

On a sheet of waxed paper or plastic wrap, shape the dough into a log about 2¹/₄ inches thick and 7 inches long. Refrigerate for 2 hours or more. Freeze for later use, if desired.

Slice the dough to a scant ¹/₄-inch thick. (These are thin cookies, if we're being true to the original!) Bake for 12 to 15 minutes, until the cookies are lightly browned; the tops will be dry. Let cool on wire racks before serving.

Chocolate Marshmallow "Scooter" Pies

brown rice flour

MAKES ABOUT 15 SANDWICH COOKIES

Inspired by the Little Debbie Chocolate Marshmallow Pies, these cookies feature two tender cookies with a marshmallow sandwiched in the middle, covered in chocolate. I daresay that these are an upscale version of the original. They are smaller, measuring 2 inches in diameter as compared to the original's 3-inch diameter. Milk chocolate chips are closer to the original, but semisweet chocolate chips make for a more interesting glaze.

$\frac{1}{3}$ cup shortening, 70 grams

$\frac{1}{2}$ cup sugar, 100 grams

$1\frac{1}{2}$ cups brown rice flour, 185 grams

1 egg

$\frac{1}{2}$ teaspoon salt

$\frac{1}{4}$ teaspoon baking soda

2 teaspoons baking powder

1 teaspoon xanthan gum

$\frac{1}{2}$ teaspoon vanilla extract

FILLING:
15 regular-size marshmallows

GLAZE:
1 cup semisweet chocolate chips, 160 grams

2 tablespoons shortening

Preheat the oven to 350°F. Lightly grease a cookie sheet.

In a medium-size bowl, combine the shortening and sugar. Beat well. Add the brown rice flour and beat well. Scrape down the sides of the mixing bowl at least once during mixing. Add the remaining batter ingredients and mix well until the dough comes together. The dough will be soft, but manageable.

Roll out the dough to $\frac{1}{8}$-inch thickness and cut it with a 2-inch circle cookie cutter. Place the slices on the prepared pan.

Bake the cookies for 9 to 10 minutes, until the edges are lightly browned. Let cool on wire racks.

(continues on next page)

| Great Fakes Cookies

For the filling, use your rolling pin to roll out each marshmallow into a circle about 2 inches in diameter.

For the glaze, combine the chocolate chips and shortening in microwave-safe cup or bowl. Microwave it on HIGH for about 2 minutes to melt, stopping to stir it periodically.

To assemble the cookies, place the marshmallow disk between two cookies and cover completely with chocolate and place on waxed paper to firm.

Note: You can refrigerate the dough for 30 minutes prior to rolling for easier handling, if desired. I just take my time and ease the cut dough from the rolling surface with a spatula.

Fig Newton-Style Cookies

brown rice flour

MAKES 32 COOKIES

I wanted to find an easy way to make this cookie yet stay true to the flavor of the famous ones found in your local grocery store. These are a little sweeter in filling and the crust is a bit more pastrylike. A very good cookie.

$^{1}/_{3}$ cup shortening, 70 grams

$1^{3}/_{4}$ cups brown rice flour, 220 grams

$^{1}/_{4}$ cup corn syrup, 80 grams

1 egg

$^{1}/_{4}$ cup sugar, 50 grams

$^{1}/_{4}$ teaspoon baking soda

1 teaspoon baking powder

$^{1}/_{2}$ teaspoon salt

1 teaspoon vanilla extract

$1^{1}/_{2}$ teaspoons xanthan gum

FILLING:

8 ounces dried figs, chopped finely

$^{1}/_{2}$ cup apple jelly, 135 grams

$^{1}/_{2}$ cup water

Preheat the oven to 350°F. Lightly grease a cookie sheet.

To make the dough, combine the shortening and brown rice flour in a medium-size bowl. Beat well. Scrape down the sides of the mixing bowl at least once during mixing. Add the remaining batter ingredients and mix well. The cookie dough will be quite heavy in texture. Once the dough comes together, continue beating for an additional minute or so to make the dough easier to handle. At this point, the dough will be very soft and should be refrigerated for at least 30 minutes.

For the filling, combine the figs, apple jelly, and water in a small saucepan over low heat. Puree it with a stick blender and continue cooking until a thick paste remains, about 1 cup of filling. Set it aside to cool.

(continues on next page)

Roll a quarter of the dough into a 5 by 8-inch rectangle. Spread ¼ cup of filling on the center third of the dough. Fold the two other thirds over the top to fully wrap the filling with dough. Place each cookie seam side down on the prepared pan. Do the same with the remaining dough.

Bake for 15 to 20 minutes until golden brown. Let cool completely on wire racks before slicing into 1-inch cookies.

Girl Scout Do-Si-Dos–Style Cookies

sorghum flour

MAKES ABOUT 24 SANDWICH COOKIES

It is strange how one peanut butter cookie can have such nuances when compared to others. In these, the base cookies are soft in peanut butter flavor and almost crackerlike in texture. The cream filling is very flavorful and spread quite thinly. The combination is delicious—it is no wonder they are so popular.

1/4 cup peanut butter, 65 grams

2 tablespoons oil, 20 grams

1/2 cup sugar, 100 grams

1 cup sorghum flour, 135 grams

1 egg

1/4 teaspoon baking soda

1/2 teaspoon salt

1/2 teaspoon xanthan gum

1/2 teaspoon vanilla extract

1 tablespoon water

FILLING:

1/4 cup confectioners' sugar, 30 grams

1/4 cup peanut butter, 65 grams

Preheat the oven to 350°F. Lightly grease a cookie sheet.

In a medium-size bowl, combine the peanut butter, oil, and sugar. Beat well. Add the sorghum flour and beat well. Scrape down the sides of the mixing bowl at least once during mixing. Add the remaining batter ingredients and mix well. Continue beating until the dough comes together; it will be oily, yet seem a little dry.

Roll scant teaspoonfuls of dough into balls about 1/2-inch in diameter and drop them onto the prepared pan. Press to no more than 1/4-inch thickness, using the bottom of a glass or butter press. Bake for 8 minutes, until the cookies just begin to brown. Let cool on wire racks.

(continues on next page)

| Great Fakes Cookies

For the filling, combine the confectioners' sugar and peanut butter. Beat until fully combined. The cream filling will be stiff and almost dry. Place a marble-size bit of creamy filling between two cookies (bottom sides facing) and press together to form a sandwich. Repeat to make the other sandwiches.

Girl Scout Lemon Chalet Cremes–Style Cookies

brown rice flour

MAKES ABOUT 25 SANDWICH COOKIES

✺

Amazingly, this little lemon sandwich cookie does not start with two lemon-flavored cookies. They taste slightly of lemon and a little cinnamon. But the filling is very lemony.

1/3 cup shortening, 70 grams

1/2 cup sugar, 100 grams

1 1/2 cup brown rice flour, 185 grams

2 egg whites

1/2 teaspoon salt

1/4 teaspoon baking soda

1 1/2 teaspoons xanthan gum

1/2 teaspoon lemon extract

1/2 teaspoon ground cinnamon

FILLING:

1/3 cup shortening, 70 grams

1 teaspoon lemon extract

3/4 cup confectioners' sugar, 90 grams

Several drops yellow food coloring (optional)

Preheat the oven to 350°F. Lightly grease a cookie sheet.

In a medium-size bowl, combine the shortening and sugar. Beat well. Add the brown rice flour and beat well. Scrape down the sides of the mixing bowl at least once during mixing. Add the remaining batter ingredients and mix well until the dough comes together; it will be very soft, yet manageable. The dough may be refrigerated for 30 minutes, for easier rolling.

Roll out the dough to a 1/8-inch thickness and cut it with a 1 1/2-inch cookie cutter. Place the cutouts on the prepared pan and press them with a butter press, or make a pretty pattern with the tines of a fork.

Bake the cookies for about 12 minutes, until lightly browned. Let cool on wire racks.

For the filling, combine all ingredients and mix until creamy. Place a marble-size bit of creamy filling between two cookies (bottom sides facing) and press together to form a sandwich. Repeat to make the other sandwiches.

Girl Scout Samoas-Style Cookies

brown rice flour

MAKES ABOUT 45 COOKIES

Duplicating the essence of this cookie was not the easiest task. But knowing that Samoas are one of the top-selling Girl Scout cookies made me plunge forward anyway. The components are a hard, sweet, little wreath-shaped cookie, heavily vanilla flavored, with an indentation down the middle. It's covered with a sticky caramel sauce, finely cut toasted coconut, and a drizzle of very sweet chocolate that's striped over the front and totally covers the base. For those of you that are still with me . . . let's make all of the components and then combine to make a very tasty, even more tender version of this fabulous cookie.

¹⁄₃ cup shortening, 70 grams

1¹⁄₂ cups brown rice flour, 185 grams

¹⁄₂ cup sugar, 100 grams

1 egg

¹⁄₄ teaspoon baking soda

¹⁄₂ teaspoon salt

1 teaspoon xanthan gum

2 teaspoons vanilla extract

Preheat the oven to 350°F. Lightly grease a cookie sheet.

In a medium-size bowl, combine the shortening and brown rice flour. Beat well. Add the remaining batter ingredients and beat well. Continue beating until the dough comes together; it will be soft like play dough.

Roll out the dough to ¹⁄₄-inch thickness. Use a 2-inch cutter for the outside of the circle and use a 1¹⁄₂-inch round cookie cutter to cut away the inside of the cookie, forming a wreath shape. Place the cookies on the prepared pan. Make a narrow indentation across the center of the wreath. This trench will eventually be filled with caramel sauce. (I used two coins—nickels—held together to

CARAMEL FILLING:
2 cups heavy whipping cream (unwhipped)

2 teaspoons vanilla extract

$3/_4$ teaspoon xanthan gum

2 cups sugar, 400 grams

TOASTED COCONUT:
2 cups sweetened flaked coconut (200 grams)

CHOCOLATE COATING:
12 ounces broken milk chocolate bars, 340 grams

$1/_4$ cup confectioners' sugar

achieve the right thickness. A board game checker may also work. Please wash this item well before using—or wrap in foil—and overlook the nonkitchen aspect of the tool.) Then prick the center of the cookie trench to help it retain its shape. Bake the cookies for 7 to 8 minutes, until the edges just begin to brown. The cookies should be crisp upon cooling. Let cool on wire racks before proceeding. Keep the oven heated to 350°F for toasting the coconut.

To make the caramel sauce, mix the cream, vanilla, and xanthan gum in a small cup. Set aside. Place the sugar in a metal saucepan and heat over high heat. Cook it until it is melted and golden brown in color. *Do not* touch the hot sugar or caramel with wooden or plastic utensils or your fingers. It will be dangerously hot. With *great caution*, immediately pour all of the cream mixture into the saucepan and stir well using a metal utensil. Bring the mixture to a boil. Remove it from the heat and continue stirring until any large pieces of cooked sugar are dissolved. Let cool. The mixture will continue to thicken during cooling.

I Great Fakes Cookies

(*continues on next page*)

To make the toasted coconut, place the coconut on a cutting board and chop it into very small pieces. (I like to "walk" the knife through the coconut. This only takes a minute or so to complete.) Spread it onto an ungreased baking sheet and place in a 350°F oven. Stir it after 3 minutes, to prevent burning. The coconut will be lightly browned when toasted for 6 to 7 minutes. Set it aside to cool.

For the drizzled and dipped chocolate coating, I suggest making two batches of coating (using half of the ingredients at a time) so that it will not harden before you have used it all. Place half the chocolate into a microwave-safe bowl and heat on HIGH for 1 to 2 minutes, until melted. Stir in half the sugar, until creamy.

To assemble the cookies, dip or spread a cookie base with melted chocolate to fully cover the base. Place it on waxed paper. Then overfill the cookie trench with caramel sauce (place the sauce in zip-type plastic bag and snip the corner) and spread it over the sides of the cookie with a knife. Sprinkle liberally with toasted coconut and press it into the underlying caramel. Allow to cool thoroughly. Peel the cookies off the waxed paper and transfer them to a clean sheet of waxed paper, shaking off the excess coconut.

Finally, prepare the remaining chocolate topping, and place it into a zip-type plastic bag and snip the corner. Pipe thin chocolate stripes across the tops of the cookies. Allow the cookies to cool again.

Note: If you lose your spunk after making twenty or thirty of these, please know that the extra dough can be used to make good sugar cookies. Just roll and bake (about 8 minutes).

| The Ultimate Gluten-Free Cookie Book

Girl Scout Tagalongs-Style Cookies

brown rice flour

MAKES ABOUT 40 COOKIES

In the original Tagalongs, the underlying cookie is rather thin, a little hard, high in vanilla flavor, and not too sweet. The peanut butter is plain and the chocolate coating is sweet. It combines for a delicious cookie that you may have enjoyed prior to dietary restriction.

1/3 cup shortening, 70 grams

1 1/2 cups brown rice flour, 185 grams

1/4 cup sugar, 50 grams

1 egg

1/4 teaspoon baking soda

1 teaspoon baking powder

1/2 teaspoon salt

1 teaspoon xanthan gum

2 teaspoons vanilla extract

CHOCOLATE COATING:
12 ounces broken milk chocolate bars, 340 grams

2 tablespoons confectioners' sugar

FILLING:
1/2 cup peanut butter

Preheat the oven to 350°F. Lightly grease a cookie sheet.

In a medium-size bowl, combine the shortening and brown rice flour. Beat well. Scrape down the sides of the mixing bowl at least once during mixing. Add the remaining ingredients and beat well. Continue beating until the dough comes together; it will be soft like play dough.

Roll out the dough to 1/8-inch thickness. Use a 1 1/2-inch round cookie cutter to cut the cookies and place them on the prepared pan. Depress the center of each cookie a bit with the back of a measuring spoon; this will eventually help hold the peanut butter. Then prick the center of the cookie to help the bottom of the cookie stay flat. Bake for 8 to 9 minutes, until the edges begin to brown. The cookies should be crisp upon cooling. Let cool well before proceeding.

I Great Fakes Cookies

(continues on next page)

For the chocolate coating, I suggest making two batches of coating (using half of the ingredients at a time) so that it does not harden before you have used it all. Place half the chocolate into a microwave-safe bowl and cook on HIGH for 1 to 2 minutes, until melted. Stir in half the sugar. Stir until creamy.

Place about ½ teaspoon of peanut butter on top of each cookie and spread, leaving a margin of ¼ to ⅓ inch from the edge of the cookie. Dip the cookies into the chocolate coating (remove the excess, especially from the bottom) and place on waxed paper to cool. The coating should be as thin as possible to mimic the original.

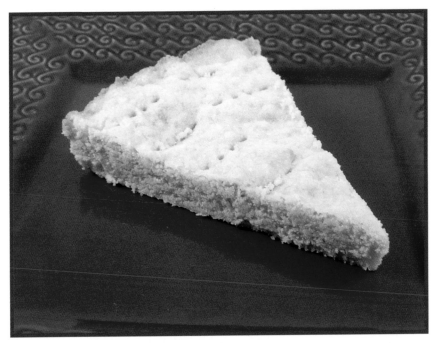

Shortbread, page 57

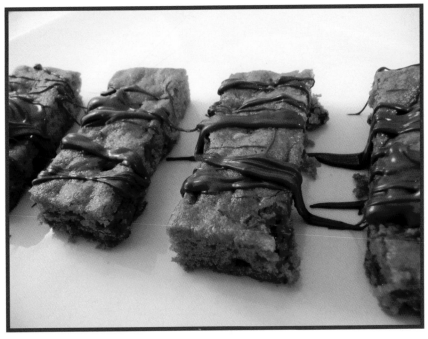

Blondies #2, page 45

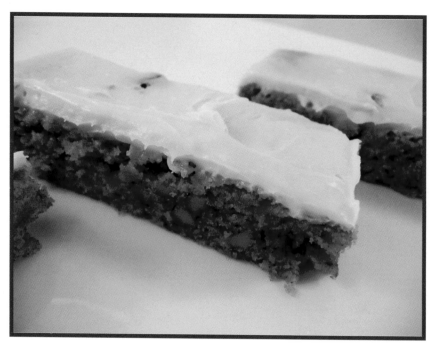

Carrot Cake Bars, page 46

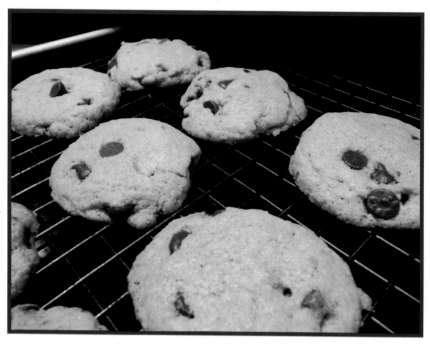

Chocolate Chip Cookies #2, page 25

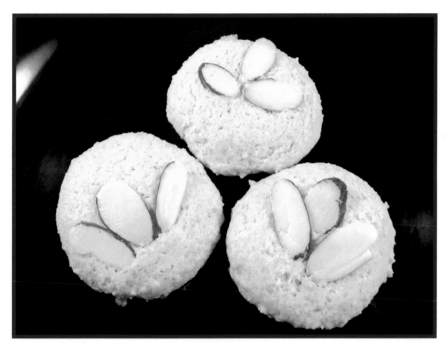

Almond Flower Cookies, page 20

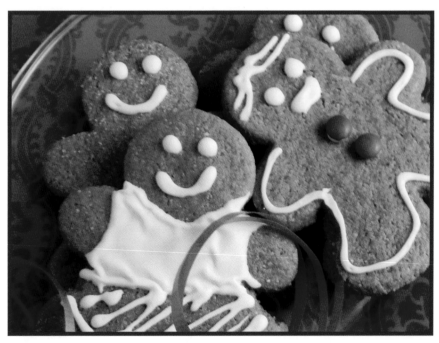

Gingerbread Men, page 81

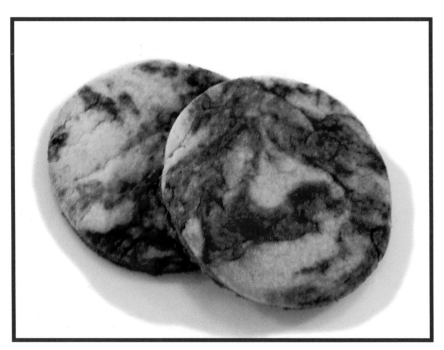

Chinese Marble Cookies, page 70

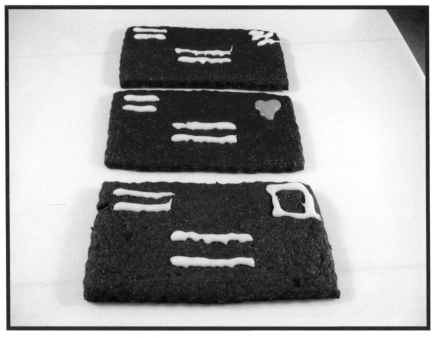

Love Letter Rolled Chocolate Sugar Cookies, page 172

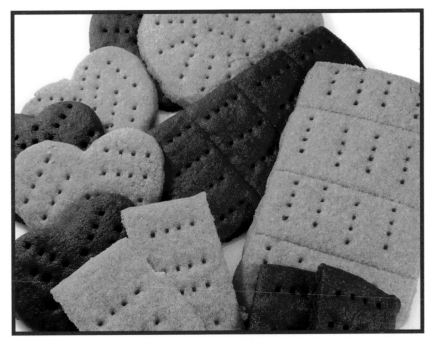

Graham Crackers, page 82

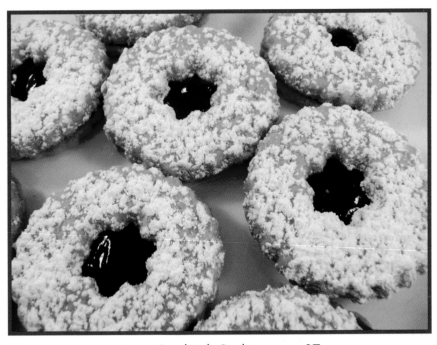

Linzer Sandwich Cookies, page 87

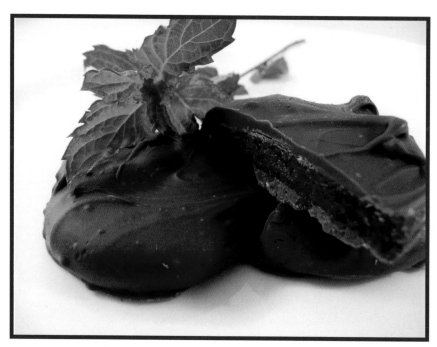

Girl Scout Thin Mints–Style Cookies, page 107

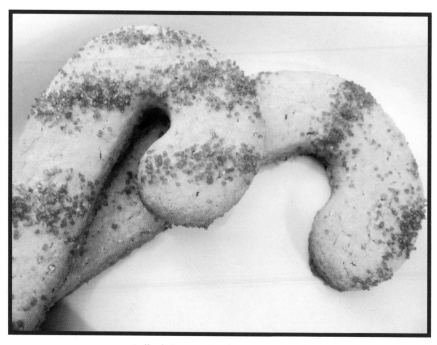

Rolled Sugar Cookies, page 89

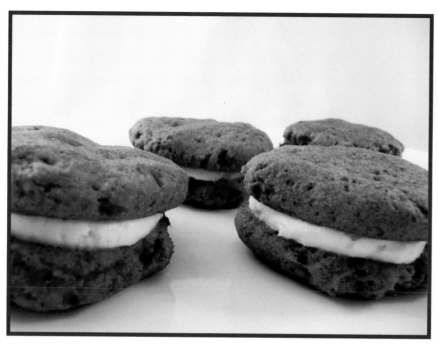

Pumpkin Sandwich Cookies (Scooter Pies), page136

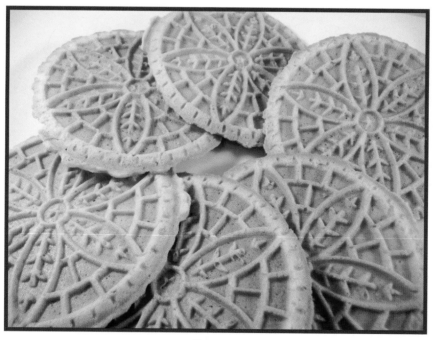

Pizzelle, page 133

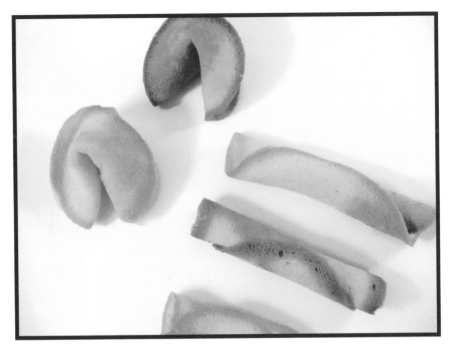

Fortune Cookies and Pirouettes, page 169

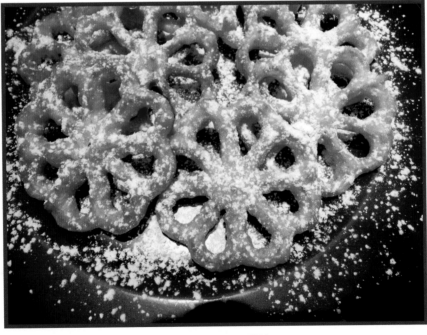

Rosettes, page 176

Girl Scout Thin Mints-Style Cookies

brown rice flour
MAKES ABOUT 25 COOKIES

In the original Thin Mints cookies, the underlying chocolate cookie is quite thin, not too sweet, and rather compact. It is the thin milk chocolate covering that is very minty.

1/3 cup oil, 65 grams

1/4 cup sugar, 50 grams

1 cup brown rice flour, 125 grams

1/3 cup unsweetened cocoa powder, 30 grams

1 egg

1/8 teaspoon baking soda

1/2 teaspoon salt

1 teaspoon xanthan gum

1 teaspoon vanilla extract

CHOCOLATE COATING:
12 ounces broken milk chocolate bars, 340 grams

2 tablespoons confectioners' sugar

1/2 teaspoon mint extract

Preheat the oven to 350°F. Lightly grease a cookie sheet.

In a medium-size bowl, combine the oil and sugar. Beat well. Add the brown rice flour and beat well. Scrape down the sides of the mixing bowl at least once during mixing. Add the remaining batter ingredients and beat well. Continue beating until the dough comes together; it will be soft and oily to the touch.

Roll out the dough to 1/8-inch thickness. Use a 1 1/2-inch round cookie cutter to cut the cookies and place them on the prepared pan. Bake the cookies for 8 to 9 minutes, until the tops are dry. Let cool well before coating; the cookies should be crisp upon cooling.

(continues on next page)

For the chocolate coating, I suggest making two batches of coating (using half of the ingredients at a time) so that it does not harden before you have used it all. Place half the chocolate into a microwave-safe bowl and cook on HIGH for 1 to 2 minutes, until melted. Stir in half the sugar and half the mint extract. Stir until creamy. Dip the cookies into the chocolate and place on waxed paper to cool. The coating should be as thin as possible to mimic the original.

Note: Milk chocolate bars melt "thinner" than do milk chocolate chips. Milk chocolate chips may be used, but will make for a thicker chocolate coating.

Girl Scout Trefoils–Style Cookies

brown rice flour

MAKES ABOUT 30 COOKIES

I realized something very interesting about the original cookies. They don't taste like a traditional shortbread. They are a little sweeter, have more vanilla flavor, and are a little smoother in texture. Besides being obviously delicious, I noted that they are like a cross between an animal cracker and traditional shortbread in flavor. I hope they bring back fond memories for you! I used an old-fashioned butter press for the design on the top. Please note that a little bit of butter makes a big flavor difference!

¹/₄ cup oil, 50 grams

2 tablespoons butter

¹/₂ cup sugar, 100 grams

1¹/₂ cups brown rice flour, 185 grams

2 egg yolks

¹/₄ teaspoon baking soda

¹/₂ teaspoon salt

1 teaspoon xanthan gum

1¹/₂ teaspoons vanilla extract

3 tablespoons water

Preheat the oven to 350°F. Lightly grease a cookie sheet.

In a medium-size bowl, combine the oil, butter, and sugar. Beat well. Add the brown rice flour and beat well. Scrape down the sides of the mixing bowl at least once during mixing. Add the remaining ingredients and beat well. Continue beating until the dough comes together.

For each cookie, shape a slightly rounded teaspoonful of dough into a ball and place it on the prepared cookie sheet. Using the bottom of a glass or a butter press that has been sprayed lightly with nonstick spray, press the ball into a circle about 1³/₄-inches wide and less than ¹/₄-inch thick.

(continues on next page)

I Great Fakes Cookies

Girl Scout Trefoils-Style Cookies *(continued)*

Bake the cookies for about 15 minutes, until the tops are lightly browned. Underbaking makes for a sugar cookie taste (which is also very good). Correct baking provides the drier cookie that is desired. Let cool on wire racks before serving.

Little Debbie Oatmeal Creme Pies–Style Cookies

oats

MAKES ABOUT 7 SANDWICH COOKIES

Unfortunately for my hips, it took quite a few cookies for me to figure this cookie out! Even duplicating the cream filling was elusive. Like the original, the oatmeal cookie is extremely soft and the filling is super sweet.

$1/2$ tablespoon raisins, 5 grams

$1^1/4$ cups rolled oats, 125 grams

$1/3$ cup oil, 65 grams

$3/4$ cup brown sugar, 150 grams

1 egg

$1/2$ teaspoon salt

$1/2$ teaspoon xanthan gum

1 teaspoon vanilla extract

1 tablespoon water

FILLING:

$1/3$ cup shortening, 70 grams

$3/4$ cup confectioners' sugar, 90 grams

$1/2$ cup marshmallow cream, 50 grams

Preheat the oven to 350°F. Lightly grease a cookie sheet.

Finely mince the raisins; using a little bit of oats mixed with the raisins will make this much easier. Place the raisins and oats in a blender. Process until most of the oats are powdery, yet a good amount of small pieces remain.

Pour the oat mixture in a mixing bowl. Add the remaining batter ingredients and mix well. A sticky-looking dough will form. Scrape down the sides of the mixing bowl at least once during mixing.

Place tablespoonfuls of dough on the prepared pan and, using moistened fingertips, press down to $1/4$-inch thickness.

(continues on next page)

Bake the cookies for 8 to 10 minutes, until the edges are lightly browned. Keep the cookies on the pan for a minute to "set" before transferring to a cooling rack. The cookies will be very pliable.

For the filling, combine the shortening and confectioners' sugar and mix until creamy. Add the marshmallow cream and mix well. Spread the bottom of one cookie with the filling and press it together with the bottom of another cookie. Repeat to make the other sandwiches.

Maple Leaf Cookies

brown rice flour

MAKES ABOUT 15 SANDWICH COOKIES

Inspired by the Maple Leaf Cookies at Trader Joe's, these cookies have a creamy center that is so full of maple flavor that it seems as if the entire cookie has maple syrup in it. Like the original, it is an understated, plain, hard vanilla cookie on the outside. For a slightly healthier cookie, omit the filling and use maple flavoring in the base cookie. Very enjoyable!

⅓ cup shortening, 70 grams

½ cup sugar, 100 grams

1½ cups brown rice flour, 185 grams

2 egg whites

½ teaspoon salt

¼ teaspoon baking soda

1½ teaspoons xanthan gum

½ teaspoon vanilla extract

FILLING:

⅓ cup shortening, 70 grams

1 teaspoon maple flavoring

¾ cup confectioners' sugar, 90 grams

Note: Roll these cookies as thinly as possible, as they do rise just a little in the oven. Also, you can refrigerate the dough for 30 minutes for easier handling, if desired. I just take my time and ease the cut dough from the rolling surface with a spatula.

Preheat the oven to 350°F. Lightly grease a cookie sheet.

In a medium-size bowl, combine the shortening and sugar. Beat well. Add the brown rice flour and beat well. Scrape down the sides of the mixing bowl at least once during mixing. Add the remaining batter ingredients and mix well until the dough comes together. The dough will be very soft, yet manageable.

Roll out the dough to ⅛-inch thickness and cut it with maple leaf–shaped cookie cutters (symmetrical for sandwiching!) or other preferred cookie cutter. Place them on the prepared pan.

Bake the cookies for about 13 minutes, until lightly browned. Let cool on wire racks.

For the filling, combine all ingredients and mix until creamy. Place a marble-size bit of creamy filling between two cookies (bottom sides facing) and press them together to form a sandwich. Repeat to make the other sandwiches.

Nutter Butter–Style Peanut Butter Sandwich Cookies

brown rice flour and cornstarch
MAKES ABOUT 15 SANDWICH COOKIES

A bent 2½-inch circle cookie cutter does a pretty good imitation of the peanut shape of these cookies. I prepared these cookies on the first day of school, which left me all alone in my kitchen. I had no one to share the excitement of a nearly perfect cookie. Dancing alone in my house was good, but these cookies are better than that!

¼ cup creamy peanut butter, 65 grams

2 tablespoons oil, 20 grams

½ cup sugar, 100 grams

1 cup brown rice flour, 125 grams

⅓ cup cornstarch, 40 grams

2 egg yolks

¼ teaspoon baking soda

½ teaspoon salt

1 teaspoon xanthan gum

1 teaspoon vanilla extract

2½ tablespoons water

FILLING:
6 tablespoons peanut butter, 100 grams

½ cup confectioners' sugar, 60 grams

¼ teaspoon vanilla extract

A few drops of water (only if needed)

Preheat the oven to 350°F. Lightly grease a cookie sheet.

In a medium-size bowl, combine the peanut butter, oil, and sugar. Beat well. Add the brown rice flour and cornstarch and beat well. Scrape down the sides of the mixing bowl at least once during mixing. Add the remaining batter ingredients and beat well until the dough almost comes together. The dough will hold together when pressed in the hand and will be oily to the touch.

Roll out the dough to ⅛-inch thickness. Use the back of a fork to crisscross wavy indentations (to mimic peanut texture). Use a 2-inch round or a cookie cutter bent into a peanut shape to cut the cookies. The dough is very easy to work with, but quite soft. Place the cutouts on the prepared pan.

Bake the cookies for 10 to 12 minutes, until the edges just begin to brown. Let cool on wire racks.

To prepare the filling, combine the peanut butter, confectioners' sugar, and vanilla. Mix until creamy. Add a few drops of water, if necessary, to the mixture. Spread the bottom of one cookie with a little filling and press it together with the bottom of another cookie. Repeat to make the other sandwiches.

Oreos-Style Cookies

brown rice flour

MAKES ABOUT 25 SANDWICH COOKIES

An original Oreo is very sweet and very chocolaty; these are, too. Grab a glass of milk for dunking. I used a decorative fondant punch set from Wilton to make pretty designs on the tops of the cookies, but a simple design can be drawn with a toothpick or the tines of a fork as well.

$^1/_3$ cup oil, 65 grams

$^1/_2$ cup sugar, 100 grams

1 cup brown rice flour, 125 grams

$^1/_3$ cup unsweetened cocoa powder, 30 grams

1 egg

$^1/_4$ teaspoon baking soda

$^1/_2$ teaspoon salt

1 teaspoon xanthan gum

1 teaspoon vanilla extract

1 tablespoon water

FILLING:

$^1/_3$ cup shortening, 70 grams

$^1/_2$ teaspoon vanilla extract

$^3/_4$ cup confectioners' sugar, 90 grams

Preheat the oven to 350°F. Lightly grease a cookie sheet.

In a medium-size bowl, combine the oil and sugar. Beat well. Add the brown rice flour and beat well. Scrape down the sides of the mixing bowl at least once during mixing. Add the remaining batter ingredients and beat well. Continue beating until the dough comes together; it will be soft and oily to the touch.

Roll out the dough to $^1/_8$-inch thickness. Use a $1^1/_2$-inch round cookie cutter to cut the cookies. Place them on the prepared pan and press the tops with a decorative stamp if you have one.

Bake the cookies for 10 minutes, until the tops are dry. The cookies should be crisp upon cooling. Let cool on wire racks.

For the filling, combine all ingredients and mix until creamy. Place a marble-size bit of creamy filling between two cookies (bottom sides facing) and press together to form a sandwich. Repeat to make the other sandwiches.

Pecan Sandies-Style Cookies

brown rice flour and pecan meal

MAKES ABOUT 25 COOKIES

Although I prefer traditional shortbread with butter, we are duplicating these famous cookie-aisle cookies, so I stay true to the flavor by using shortening instead. If you loved the Keebler cookie, you will love these, too. (But if you want to use butter, substitute ⅓ cup butter for the shortening, decrease the water to 2 teaspoons, and increase the xanthan gum to 1⅓ teaspoons.)

⅓ cup shortening, 70 grams

½ cup sugar, 100 grams

1¼ cups brown rice flour, 220 grams

¼ cup pecan meal, 20 grams (or substitute ¼ cup brown rice flour)

1 egg

2 teaspoons baking powder

¼ teaspoon baking soda

½ teaspoon salt

1 teaspoon xanthan gum

½ teaspoon vanilla extract

1 tablespoon water

½ cup chopped pecans

When ready to bake, preheat the oven to 350°F. Lightly grease a cookie sheet.

In a medium-size bowl, combine the shortening and sugar. Beat well. Add the brown rice flour and mix well. Scrape down the sides of the mixing bowl at least once during mixing. Add the remaining ingredients, except for the pecan pieces, and mix well. The cookie dough will form large clumps, but will not quite come together to form a ball; this is okay. Add the chopped pecans and mix well.

On a sheet of waxed paper or plastic wrap, shape the dough into a log about 2 inches thick and 7½-inches long. Refrigerate for 2 hours or more. You can also freeze for later use, if desired.

Slice the dough into ¼-inch slices and place on the prepared pan. Bake the cookies for about 15 minutes, until they are lightly browned around the edges and the tops are dry. Let cool on wire racks before serving.

Pepperidge Farm Milano-Style Cookies

brown rice flour

MAKES ABOUT 18 SANDWICH COOKIES

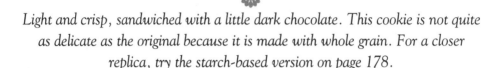

Light and crisp, sandwiched with a little dark chocolate. This cookie is not quite as delicate as the original because it is made with whole grain. For a closer replica, try the starch-based version on page 178.

1/3 cup oil, 65 grams

1/3 cup sugar, 75 grams

1 cup brown rice flour, 125 grams

1 egg, plus 1 egg white

1/4 teaspoon baking soda

1/2 teaspoon salt

1/2 teaspoon xanthan gum

1/2 teaspoon vanilla extract

FILLING:
4 ounces broken dark chocolate
    bar

Preheat the oven to 325°F. Lightly grease a cookie sheet.

In a medium-size bowl, combine oil and sugar. Beat well. Add the brown rice flour and beat well. Scrape down the sides of the mixing bowl at least once during mixing. Add the remaining ingredients and mix well. The dough will be a thick, cakelike batter.

Place the batter into a zip-type plastic bag. Cut off one corner at a 1/3-inch angle. Pipe 2- to 2 1/2-inch-long fingers well apart onto the prepared pan. The cookies will spread during baking.

Bake for 10 to 12 minutes, until the edges of the cookies are very golden. (Underbake and the cookies will not be crisp throughout—but still tasty!) Let cool on wire racks.

Place the chocolate into a microwave-safe bowl and heat on HIGH for 1 to 2 minutes, until melted. Spread the bottom of one cookie with the melted chocolate and press it together with the bottom of another cookie. Repeat to make the other sandwiches.

Pepperidge Farm White Chocolate Macadamia Crispy-Style Cookies

brown rice flour

MAKES ABOUT 22 COOKIES

A big, sweet, crispy, tender cookie, with white chocolate chunks and macadamia nuts (our version has a little extra). Note the lower baking temperature, which is necessary for the center to cook before the edges burn.

¼ cup butter, 55 grams

¼ cup oil, 50 grams

½ cup plus 2 tablespoons sugar, 125 grams

1½ cups brown rice flour, 185 grams

1 egg, plus 1 egg yolk

¼ teaspoon baking soda

1 teaspoon baking powder

½ teaspoon salt

1 teaspoon xanthan gum

1 teaspoon vanilla extract

⅓ cup roughly chopped macadamia nuts, 50 grams

⅓ cup roughly chopped white chocolate chips, 60 grams

Preheat the oven to 325°F. Very lightly grease a cookie sheet.

In a medium-size bowl, combine the butter, oil, and sugar. Beat well. Add the flour and beat well. Scrape down the sides of the mixing bowl at least once during mixing. Add the remaining batter ingredients and beat well. Continue beating until the dough comes together; it will be soft and almost creamy. Set aside.

Drop rounded tablespoonfuls of the dough onto the prepared pan. Press to ¼-inch thickness. Bake the cookies for 10 to 12 minutes, until the edges begin to brown. Let cool on wire racks before serving.

7

Sandwich, Shaped, and Filled Cookies

This chapter is an eclectic mix of unique cookies. From deep-fried Rosettes and nicely pressed Pizzelle to picture-perfect Thumbprint Cookies, you will be cookie-ready for nearly any occasion.

Among my favorites are the Chocolate-Cherry Cookies and the classic Snickerdoodles. The Almond Biscotti is a great coffeetime treat and all of the sandwich cookies are soft and tender with a tasty creamy filling.

Almond Biscotti

brown rice flour
MAKES ABOUT 30 COOKIES

This recipe is fashioned after the mini biscotti at Trader Joe's. Almond and butter team up for a delicious cookie.

$\frac{1}{3}$ cup butter, 70 grams

$\frac{1}{3}$ cup sugar, 75 grams

$1\frac{1}{2}$ cups brown rice flour, 185 grams

2 eggs

$\frac{1}{4}$ teaspoon baking soda

2 teaspoons baking powder

$\frac{1}{2}$ teaspoon salt

1 teaspoon xanthan gum

$1\frac{1}{2}$ teaspoons almond extract

$\frac{1}{2}$ cup sliced almonds

Preheat the oven to 350°F. Lightly grease a cookie sheet.

In a medium-size bowl, combine the butter and sugar. Beat well. Add the brown rice flour and mix well. Scrape down the sides of the mixing bowl at least once during mixing. Add the remaining ingredients and mix well. The dough will be soft and heavy.

Shape about half the dough into a flattened log about ½-inch thick and place on the prepared pan. Do the same with the other half of the dough.

Bake the logs for 20 minutes. Let cool completely on wire racks. Cut each log into slices about ½-inch thick and place these back on the prepared pan. Bake the biscotti for an additional 10 to 15 minutes until quite dry. Let cool again on wire racks before serving

Chocolate-Cherry Cookies

brown rice flour

MAKES ABOUT 27 COOKIES

This recipe is my gluten-free re-creation of the Chocolate Cherry Cookies contained in the 100 Best Cookies by Better Homes and Gardens. They taste like a rich chocolate cookie crossed with a cherry cordial. Delicious.

$\frac{1}{3}$ cup oil, 65 grams

$\frac{1}{2}$ cup sugar, 100 grams

1 cup brown rice flour, 125 grams

$\frac{1}{3}$ cup unsweetened cocoa powder, 30 grams

2 eggs

$\frac{1}{4}$ teaspoon baking soda

1 teaspoon baking powder

$\frac{1}{2}$ teaspoon salt

$\frac{1}{2}$ teaspoon xanthan gum

1 teaspoon vanilla extract

TOPPINGS:

1 (10-ounce) jar maraschino cherries

1 cup chocolate chips

$\frac{1}{2}$ cup sweetened condensed milk

Preheat the oven to 350°F. Lightly grease a cookie sheet.

In a medium-size bowl, combine the oil and sugar. Beat well. Add the brown rice flour and beat well. Scrape down the sides of the mixing bowl at least once during mixing. Add the remaining batter ingredients and beat well. Continue beating until the dough comes together; it will be very soft.

Drop rounded teaspoonfuls of the dough onto the prepared pan. With moistened fingertips, press the dough to $\frac{1}{3}$-inch thickness and make a depression in the middle, using your fingertip.

Place a cherry (stem removed) in the hollowed-out middle of each unbaked cookie. Save the cherry juice!

(continues on next page)

| Sandwich, Shaped, and Filled Cookies

In a microwave-safe cup, combine 1½ table-spoons of the cherry juice, the chocolate chips, and the condensed milk. Microwave on HIGH for 1½ to 2 minutes, stirring frequently, until the chocolate melts and is of spreading consistency. (The topping may be thinned with additional cherry juice if necessary.) Drop a rounded teaspoonful of the chocolate mixture over each cherry to cover. (This will seem like a large amount.) It is important to fully cover the cherry.

Bake the cookies for about 10 minutes, until the edges are dry. Let cool on wire racks before serving.

Chocolate Crinkles

brown rice flour
MAKES ABOUT 25 COOKIES

*A very chocolaty cookie, covered with confectioners' sugar, then baked.
This cookie is a favorite of my older son.*

$^1/_3$ cup oil, 65 grams

$^1/_2$ cup sugar, 100 grams

1 cup brown rice flour, 125 grams

$^1/_3$ cup unsweetened cocoa
powder, 30 grams

2 eggs

$^1/_4$ teaspoon baking soda

1 teaspoon baking powder

$^1/_2$ teaspoon salt

$^1/_2$ teaspoon xanthan gum

1 teaspoon vanilla extract

$^1/_4$ cup confectioners' sugar,
30 grams

Preheat the oven to 350°F. Lightly grease a cookie sheet.

In a medium-size bowl, combine the oil and sugar. Beat well. Add the brown rice flour and beat well. Scrape down the sides of the mixing bowl at least once during mixing. Add the remaining ingredients and beat well. Continue beating until the dough comes together; it will be very soft.

Drop rounded teaspoonfuls of the dough into the confectioners' sugar (or shape the dough into small balls and drop them in) and gently cover them with confectioners' sugar. Place them on the prepared pan and press the dough balls down to $^1/_4$-inch thickness. (This step is very important.)

Bake the cookies for 10 minutes, until dry. Let cool on wire racks before serving.

Note: A heavy hand in applying the confectioners' sugar makes for a more visible crinkle to the cookie.

Chocolate-Mint Sandwich Cookies

sorghum flour

MAKES ABOUT 24 SANDWICH COOKIES

Much like the popular Oreo, these cookies have that predictable creamy filling, but the cookie is just a bit crisper and minty!

1/3 cup oil, 65 grams

1/2 cup sugar, 100 grams

1 cup sorghum flour, 135 grams

1/3 cup unsweetened cocoa powder, 30 grams

1 egg

1/4 teaspoon baking soda

1/2 teaspoon salt

1/2 teaspoon xanthan gum

1 teaspoon mint extract

FILLING:

1/3 cup shortening, 70 grams

1/2 teaspoon vanilla extract

3/4 cup confectioners' sugar, 90 grams

Preheat the oven to 350°F. Lightly grease a cookie sheet.

In a medium-size bowl, combine the oil and sugar. Beat well. Add the sorghum flour and beat well. Scrape down the sides of the mixing bowl at least once during mixing. Add the remaining batter ingredients and beat well. Continue beating until the dough comes together. The dough will be oily and dry at the same time.

Roll out the dough to 1/8-inch thickness. Use a 1 1/2-inch round cookie cutter to cut the cookies. Place them on the prepared pan and press the tops with a decorative stamp if you have one.

Bake the cookies for 8 minutes, until the tops are dry and lose their sheen. Let cool on wire racks.

For the filling, combine all the ingredients and mix until creamy. Place a marble-size bit of creamy filling between two cookies (bottom sides facing) and press together to form a sandwich. Repeat to make the other sandwiches.

Chocolate Sandwich Cookies (Scooter Pies)

brown rice flour

MAKES ABOUT 11 SANDWICH COOKIES

Essentially a soft, cakelike cookie with a cream cheese filling.

$^1/_3$ cup oil, 65 grams

$^3/_4$ cup sugar, 150 grams

1 cup brown rice flour, 125 grams

$^1/_3$ cup unsweetened cocoa powder, 30 grams

1 egg

$^1/_2$ cup plain yogurt, 120 grams

1 teaspoon baking soda

$^1/_2$ teaspoon salt

$^1/_2$ teaspoon xanthan gum

1 teaspoon vanilla extract

FILLING:

$^1/_3$ cup shortening, 70 grams

$^3/_4$ cup confectioners' sugar, 90 grams

4 ounces cream cheese, 110 grams

$^1/_2$ teaspoon vanilla extract

Preheat the oven to 350°F. Lightly grease a cookie sheet.

In a medium-size bowl, combine the oil and sugar. Beat well. Add the brown rice flour and beat well. Scrape down the sides of the mixing bowl at least once during mixing. Add the remaining batter ingredients and mix well; the dough will be like a thick cake batter.

Drop rounded tablespoonfuls of the dough onto the prepared pan. The cookies will spread during baking.

Bake for 9 to 10 minutes, until the cookies take on a bit of color at the edges and the tops appear dry. Let cool on wire racks.

For the filling, blend all the ingredients until light and fluffy. Place a tablespoon of the filling between two cookies (bottom sides facing) and press together to form a sandwich. Repeat to make the other sandwiches.

Filled Triangle Cookies

brown rice flour

MAKES BETWEEN 25 AND 30 COOKIES

This recipe uses the Rolled Sugar Cookie recipe, but opts to use all butter. The extra buttery flavor is nice to compliment the flavor of the jam. I chose strawberry, but any jam may be substituted.

½ cup butter, 110 grams

½ cup sugar, 100 grams

1½ cups brown rice flour, 185 grams

1 egg plus 1 egg yolk

¼ teaspoon baking soda

½ teaspoon salt

1¼ teaspoons xanthan gum

1 teaspoon vanilla extract

TOPPING:

½ cup jam

2 tablespoons confectioners' sugar

Preheat the oven to 350°F. Very lightly grease a cookie sheet.

In a medium-size bowl, combine the butter and sugar. Beat well. Add the brown rice flour and beat well. Scrape down the sides of the mixing bowl at least once during mixing. Add the remaining batter ingredients and beat well. Continue beating until the dough comes together. The dough will be too soft to roll. Refrigerate for 1 hour.

Roll out the dough to between ⅛- and ¼-inch thickness. Working with just one cookie at a time, use a cookie cutter to cut a 3-inch circle. Place the cutout on the prepared pan and place about 1 teaspoon of jam in the center of the cookie. Imagine a triangle whose points extend to the circumference of the dough. Fold the curved parts outside the triangle upward and partially over the jam.

Bring the corners of these folds together to form the three corners and pinch the edges together so the jam does not leak out. (This is much easier than it sounds.) Continue forming cookies with the remaining dough and jam until the sheet is filled.

Bake the cookies for 10 to 12 minutes, until the edges begin to brown. Let cool on wire racks. Dust with confectioners' sugar.

| Sandwich, Shaped, and Filled Cookies

Lemon Tassies

brown rice flour

MAKES BETWEEN 20 AND 24 TASSIES

Like the Pecan Tassies, this cookie is made with a very slight modification to my piecrust (rice-based) recipe in You Won't Believe It's Gluten-Free! *These cookies are great to make if you've made meringues and want to use the leftover egg yolks. They are also great to make if you just love lemon, like I do.*

4 ounces cream cheese

2 tablespoons butter

³/₄ cup brown rice flour, 95 grams

pinch of salt

1 teaspoon sugar

¹/₂ teaspoon xanthan gum

¹/₄ teaspoon baking soda

FILLING:

3 egg yolks

¹/₂ cup sugar, 100 grams

¹/₃ cup frozen lemonade concentrate, 95 grams

3 tablespoons butter, 40 grams

TOPPING (OPTIONAL):
Confectioners' sugar

Preheat the oven to 400°F. Lightly grease a 24-count mini-muffin pan.

For the tart shells, combine all the batter ingredients in a medium-size bowl and mix well until the dough comes together.

Drop rounded teaspoonfuls of the dough into the cups of the prepared pan and press the center with the back of a spoon to evenly form tart shells. Prick the bottom of the shells with a fork to discourage air pockets. Bake for about 10 minutes, until golden brown. Remove the shells from the oven and cool on wire racks.

For the filling, combine all the filling ingredients in a small saucepan and mix well. (The butter will melt during cooking.) Over medium heat and stirring constantly, bring the mixture to a boil and continue cooking for about a minute, then remove it from the heat to let cool. The mixture will thicken upon standing. Spoon the filling into the tart shells. Dust with confectioners' sugar, if desired, before serving.

Mocha Meltaways

brown rice flour

MAKES ABOUT 30 COOKIES

Another melt-in-your-mouth cookie hidden beneath a light coating of confectioners' sugar. Cocoa and coffee combine to create this delicious flavor.

⅓ cup shortening, 70 grams

½ cup sugar, 100 grams

1¼ cups brown rice flour, 155 grams

1 egg

¼ cup unsweetened cocoa powder, 20 grams

¼ teaspoon baking soda

1 teaspoon baking powder

½ teaspoon salt

1 teaspoon xanthan gum

1 teaspoon vanilla extract

1½ teaspoons instant coffee dissolved in 1 teaspoon hot water

TOPPING:
⅔ cup confectioners' sugar

Preheat the oven to 325°F. Lightly grease a cookie sheet.

In a medium-size bowl, combine shortening and sugar. Beat well. Scrape down the sides of the mixing bowl at least once during mixing. Add the brown rice flour and beat well. Add the remaining ingredients and mix well. The cookie dough will form large clumps, but will not quite come together to form a ball. Press it together with your hands.

Roll the dough into 1-inch balls, about 1 rounded teaspoonful. (Alternatively, you can roll out the dough to ⅓-inch thickness and cut it with 1-inch cookie cutters. This makes for a very pretty presentation.) Place the cookies on the prepared pan.

Bake the cookies for 12 to 15 minutes, until lightly browned. Immediately roll them in confectioners' sugar. Let cool on wire racks before serving.

Pecan Tassies

brown rice flour
MAKES BETWEEN 20 AND 24 TASSIES

This cookie is made with a very slight modification to my piecrust (rice-based) recipe in You Won't Believe It's Gluten-Free! *The filling is rich, but not too sweet.*

4 ounces cream cheese

2 tablespoons butter

³/₄ cup brown rice flour, 95 grams

Pinch of salt

1 teaspoon sugar

¹/₂ teaspoon xanthan gum

¹/₄ teaspoon baking soda

FILLING:

1 egg, plus 1 egg yolk

¹/₂ cup brown sugar, 100 grams

¹/₄ teaspoon salt

¹/₄ cup light corn syrup, 80 grams

¹/₂ teaspoon vanilla extract

¹/₄ teaspoon white vinegar

³/₄ cup chopped pecans, 65 grams

Preheat the oven to 400°F. Lightly grease a 24-count mini-muffin pan.

For the tart shells, combine all the batter ingredients in a medium-size bowl and mix well until the dough comes together.

Drop rounded teaspoonfuls of the dough into the cups of the prepared pan and press the center of each dough ball with the back of a spoon to evenly form tart shells. Place them in the hot oven for 5 minutes. Remove the pan from the oven and cool on wire racks.

Reduce the oven temperature to 350°F.

For the filling, combine all the ingredients and mix very well. Spoon the filling into the center of the shells.

Bake the cookies for about 10 minutes, until the filling is golden brown. Let cool on wire racks before serving.

Note: Corn syrup adds a gooeyness to this pie filling and that makes it the sweetener of choice to pair with the brown sugar. Also, you can fill the shells before baking them, but the filling will not be as separate.

| The Ultimate Gluten-Free Cookie Book

Pizzelle

brown rice flour
MAKES ABOUT 13 FOUR-INCH COOKIES

A pizzelle is a wonderful, crisp, extremely thin cookie made with the use of a pizzelle maker. Essentially, the machine makes two flat, circular, wafflelike cookies and is very easy to use. These cookies can be wrapped (warm) around a dowel to make cannoli shells, draped over a cup to form cookie bowls, used to make ice cream sandwiches, or simply enjoyed as is.

$1/3$ cup sugar, 75 grams

2 eggs

$1/4$ cup oil, 50 grams

1 cup brown rice flour, 125 grams

$1/4$ teaspoon baking soda

1 teaspoon baking powder

Pinch of salt

$1/2$ teaspoon xanthan gum

1 teaspoon vanilla extract

Turn on the pizzelle machine.

In a medium-size bowl, combine the sugar and eggs. Beat until light and thick, then set aside. In another bowl, combine the oil and brown rice flour and beat well. Scrape down the sides of the mixing bowl at least once during mixing. Add the remaining ingredients, including the egg sugar mixture, and beat well. The dough will thicken as you mix.

Place about 1 tablespoon of dough onto each pizzelle spot. Cook until very lightly browned (this is a $3\frac{1}{2}$ setting on my Cuisinart model). Let cool on wire racks before serving.

| Sandwich, Shaped, and Filled Cookies

Pizzelle, Almond

brown rice flour and almond meal
MAKES ABOUT 14 FOUR-INCH COOKIES

These pizzelle are perhaps the thinnest, lightest, and crispest of the ones presented here. I couldn't stop eating them! With the use of vanilla, the almond flavor is subtle. For a stronger flavor, opt for almond extract.

$1/3$ cup sugar, 75 grams

2 eggs

$1/4$ cup oil, 50 grams

$3/4$ cup brown rice flour, 95 grams

$1/4$ cup almond meal, 30 grams

$1/4$ teaspoon baking soda

1 teaspoon baking powder

Pinch of salt

$1/2$ teaspoon xanthan gum

$1/2$ teaspoon vanilla or almond extract

Turn on the pizzelle machine.

In a medium-size bowl, combine the sugar and eggs. Beat until light and thick, then set aside. In another bowl, combine the oil and brown rice flour. Beat well. Scrape down the sides of the mixing bowl at least once during mixing. Add the remaining ingredients, including the egg mixture, and beat well. The dough will thicken as you mix; it should be thick.

Place about 1 tablespoon of dough onto each pizzelle spot. Cook until very lightly browned (this is a $3\frac{1}{2}$ setting on my Cuisinart model). Let cool on wire racks before serving.

Pizzelle, Chocolate

brown rice flour

MAKES ABOUT 14 FOUR-INCH COOKIES

*If you enjoy pizzelle, please do not limit yourself to the traditional version.
I am a firm believer that chocolate makes almost everything better.
This version is not very sweet. Increase the sugar by a tablespoon or so if
you'd like a sweeter cookie.*

$1/3$ cup sugar, 75 grams

2 eggs

$1/4$ cup oil, 50 grams

$3/4$ cup brown rice flour, 95 grams

$1/4$ cup unsweetened cocoa
powder, 20 grams

$1/4$ teaspoon baking soda

$1/2$ teaspoon baking powder

Pinch of salt

$1/4$ teaspoon xanthan gum

$1/2$ teaspoon vanilla extract

Turn on the pizzelle machine.

In a medium-size bowl, combine the sugar and eggs. Beat until light and thick, then set aside. In another bowl, combine the oil and brown rice flour. Beat well. Scrape down the sides of the mixing bowl at least once during mixing. Add the remaining ingredients, including the egg mixture, and beat well. The dough will thicken as you mix.

Place about 1 tablespoon of dough onto each pizzelle spot. Cook until very lightly browned (this is a $3\frac{1}{2}$ setting on my Cuisinart model). Let cool on wire racks before serving.

Pumpkin Sandwich Cookies (Scooter Pies)

sorghum flour

MAKES ABOUT 11 SANDWICH COOKIES

✤

Are you a fan of the pumpkin cake roll that has a cream cheese filling? This soft pumpkin cookie is a cross between a whoopie pie and a pumpkin cake roll.

⅓ cup oil, 65 grams

½ cup brown sugar, 100 grams

1 cup sorghum flour, 135 grams

1 egg

½ cup canned pumpkin

1 teaspoon baking soda

½ teaspoon salt

1 teaspoon xanthan gum

1 teaspoon pumpkin pie spice

½ teaspoon vanilla extract

FILLING:

⅓ cup shortening, 70 grams

¾ cup confectioners' sugar, 90 grams

4 ounces cream cheese, 110 grams

½ teaspoon vanilla extract

Preheat the oven to 350°F. Lightly grease a cookie sheet.

In a medium-size bowl, combine the oil and sugar. Beat well. Add the sorghum flour and beat well. Scrape down the sides of the mixing bowl at least once during mixing. Add the remaining ingredients and mix well. Continue beating until the dough comes together; it will be soft and airy.

Drop rounded tablespoonfuls of the dough onto the prepared pan. Press to ¼-inch thickness with moist fingertips.

Bake for 10 minutes, until the cookies just begin to brown at the edges. Let cool on wire racks.

For the filling, blend all the ingredients until light and fluffy. Press a tablespoon of filling between two cookies (bottom sides facing) and press together to form a sandwich. Repeat to make the other sandwiches.

Red Velvet Sandwich Cookies (Scooter Pies)

brown rice flour

MAKES ABOUT 10 SANDWICH COOKIES

This is a popular sandwich cookie in my area: a soft red velvet cookie with a cream cheese filling. The flavor is hard to define . . . although it does contain cocoa, it's not chocolate.

$^1/_3$ cup oil, 65 grams

$^1/_2$ cup sugar, 100 grams

1 cup brown rice flour, 125 grams

1 tablespoon unsweetened cocoa powder

1 egg

$^1/_2$ cup plain yogurt, 120 grams

1 teaspoon baking soda

$^1/_2$ teaspoon salt

$^3/_4$ teaspoon xanthan gum

1 teaspoon vanilla extract

1 teaspoon liquid red food coloring

FILLING:

$^1/_3$ cup shortening, 70 grams

$^3/_4$ cup confectioners' sugar, 90 grams

4 ounces cream cheese, 110 grams

$^1/_2$ teaspoon vanilla extract

Preheat the oven to 350°F. Lightly grease a cookie sheet.

In a medium-size bowl, combine the oil and sugar. Beat well. Add the brown rice flour and beat well. Scrape down the sides of the mixing bowl at least once during mixing. Add the remaining batter ingredients and mix well. The dough will be a thick, cake-like batter.

Drop rounded tablespoonfuls of the dough well apart onto the prepared pan. The cookie will spread during baking.

Bake for 9 to 10 minutes, until the cookies take on a bit of color at the edges and the tops appear dry. Let cool on wire racks.

For the filling, blend all the ingredients until light and fluffy. Press a tablespoon of filling between two cookies (bottom sides facing) and press together to form a sandwich. Repeat to make the other sandwiches.

Rugalach

brown rice flour

MAKES 24 COOKIES

Creating a gluten-free dough that does not bind with a filling is difficult. Often, prebaking a shell or crust is the answer to this problem. But I had to figure out something different for rugalach. Finally, an answer bounced into my head—to use corn syrup as part of the sweetener. A brown sugar–nut–raisin filling is used here, but your favorite jam would make a great alternative!

¹/₃ cup shortening, 70 grams

1³/₄ cups brown rice flour, 220 grams

¹/₄ cup corn syrup, 80 grams

1 egg

¹/₄ cup sugar, 50 grams

¹/₄ teaspoon baking soda

1 teaspoon baking powder

¹/₂ teaspoon salt

1 teaspoon vanilla extract

1¹/₂ teaspoons xanthan gum

Preheat the oven to 350°F. Lightly grease a cookie sheet.

For the dough, in a medium-size bowl, combine the shortening and brown rice flour. Beat well. Scrape down the sides of the mixing bowl at least once during mixing. Add the remaining batter ingredients and mix well. The cookie dough will be quite heavy in texture. Once the dough comes together, continue beating it for an additional minute or so to make the dough easier to handle. It will be very soft and should be refrigerated for at least 30 minutes.

For the filling, combine all the ingredients in a small bowl and mix well. Set aside.

FILLING:

1/2 cup chopped pecans,
60 grams

1/4 cup raisins, chopped finely,
40 grams

2 tablespoons brown sugar

Divide the dough in half. Roll out each half into a 9-inch circle. Spread each circle with the filling, then cut it into twelve wedges (like pie slices). Roll each wedge into a crescent shape, rolling from the broad perimeter to the point, and place it on the prepared pan. Bake the rugalach for 15 to 20 minutes, until golden brown. Let cool on wire racks before serving.

Sandwich, Shaped, and Filled Cookies

Sand Balls

brown rice flour and almond meal
MAKES ABOUT 30 COOKIES

This recipe is inspired by a melt-in-your-mouth holiday nut ball cookie. I've used almond meal to achieve the melt-in-your-mouth texture. Although the components are simple, avoid substitution. Using butter for shortening removes the melting texture of the cookie. Other nut meals do not provide adequate dough structure. And, finally, egg is an important part of this recipe, despite not seeming correct.

1/3 cup shortening, 70 grams

1/2 cup sugar, 100 grams

1 cup brown rice flour, 125 grams

1 egg

1/2 cup almond meal, 60 grams

1/4 teaspoon baking soda

2 teaspoons baking powder

1/2 teaspoon salt

1 teaspoon xanthan gum

1 teaspoon vanilla extract

TOPPING:
2/3 cup confectioners' sugar

Preheat the oven to 325°F. Lightly grease a cookie sheet.

In a medium-size bowl, combine the shortening and sugar. Beat well. Scrape down the sides of the mixing bowl at least once during mixing. Add the brown rice flour and beat well. Add the remaining ingredients and mix well. The cookie dough will form large clumps, but will not quite come together to form a ball. Press it together with your hands.

Roll the dough into 1-inch balls, about 1 rounded teaspoonful each. Place on the prepared pan.

Bake for 12 to 15 minutes, until lightly browned. Immediately roll in confectioners' sugar. Let cool on wire racks before serving.

Snickerdoodles

brown rice flour

MAKES ABOUT 30 COOKIES

A soft, tender, buttery sugar cookie rolled in cinnamon sugar.
As a side note, this is among the prettiest doughs in this book.
Soft and very traditional in appearance.

¹/₄ cup butter, 110 grams

¹/₄ cup oil, 50 grams

¹/₂ cup sugar, 100 grams

1¹/₂ cups brown rice flour, 185 grams

1 egg plus 1 egg yolk

¹/₄ teaspoon baking soda

1 teaspoon baking powder

¹/₂ teaspoon salt

1 teaspoon xanthan gum

1 teaspoon vanilla extract

TOPPING:

³/₄ teaspoon ground cinnamon

3 tablespoons sugar

Preheat the oven to 350°F. Very lightly grease a cookie sheet.

In a medium-size bowl, combine the butter, oil, and sugar. Beat well. Add the brown rice flour and beat well. Scrape down the sides of the mixing bowl at least once during mixing. Add the remaining ingredients and beat well. Continue beating until the dough comes together. The dough will be soft and almost creamy. Set aside.

For the topping, combine the cinnamon and sugar. Mix well.

Place a rounded teaspoonful of dough in the cinnamon-sugar mixture (or gently shape into balls and place in the mixture). Gently roll the dough in the sugar mixture to cover it. Place it on the prepared pan. Press it down to ¹/₄-inch thickness.

Bake for about 10 minutes, until the edges begin to brown. Let cool on wire racks before serving.

Thumbprint Cookies

brown rice flour

MAKES ABOUT 25 COOKIES

A soft tender cookie covered with nuts and enhanced by a bit of jam.
A very nice cookie.

¹/₃ cup oil, 65 grams

¹/₂ cup sugar, 100 grams

1¹/₄ cups brown rice flour,
    155 grams

2 eggs

¹/₄ teaspoon baking soda

1 teaspoon baking powder

¹/₂ teaspoon salt

1¹/₄ teaspoons xanthan gum

1 teaspoon vanilla extract

TOPPING:
³/₄ cup very finely chopped
    pecans, 90 grams

¹/₂ cup seedless raspberry jam

Preheat the oven to 350°F. Lightly grease a cookie sheet.

In a medium-size bowl, combine the oil and sugar. Beat well. Add the brown rice flour and beat well. Scrape down the sides of the mixing bowl at least once during mixing. Add the remaining ingredients and beat well. The batter will be very thick and sticky.

Drop rounded teaspoonfuls of the dough into the nuts. Gently coat the dough balls and place them on the prepared pan. Press each down to ¹/₃-inch thickness and then press the center with your thumb to make room for the jam.

Bake for about 10 minutes, until the cookies begin to take on color. If the cookie centers are not very indented, gently them press again with your thumb. Let cool on wire racks. Place about ¹/₂ teaspoon of jam into the center of each cookie and sprinkle with nuts, if desired.

8

Egg-Free Cookies

This chapter covers the basics when it comes to making egg-free versions of your favorite cookies. (In addition to the recipes in this chapter, there are also a number of naturally egg-free recipes elsewhere in this book, including the Trail Mix Bars and Rice Cereal Bars.) For simplicity, I opted to avoid egg substitutes and the sometimes recommended flaxseed alternative. To retain the moistness and texture of these cookies, I simply used honey or corn syrup as the primary sweetener. Applesauce, bananas, and pumpkin are also naturals in the egg-free baking pantry.

As a side note, honey is sweeter than corn syrup in baking. And corn syrup gives a bit of hardness to the exterior of a cookie. Corn syrup also provides a neutral flavor base for certain cookies.

Egg-free baking doesn't have to be very different from traditional baking. It only takes ordinary ingredients to benefit this special dietary need.

Almond Joy–Style Cookies

cornstarch or potato starch

MAKES ABOUT 20 COOKIES

*This cookie is inspired by the Almond Joy candy bar. They require few
ingredients and will satisfy any sweet tooth!*

1 (7-ounce) bag sweetened
flaked coconut (2²/₃ cups)

2 tablespoons cornstarch or
potato starch

¹/₂ cup sweetened condensed milk

About 20 almonds

CHOCOLATE COATING:
12 ounces broken milk chocolate
bars, 340 grams

¹/₂ teaspoon vanilla extract

Preheat oven to 325°F. Lightly grease a mini-muffin pan.

In a medium-size bowl, combine the coconut, cornstarch, and condensed milk. Beat very well.

Drop rounded teaspoonfuls of the dough into each cup of the muffin pan. Top each cookie with an almond.

Bake the cookies for 13 to 15 minutes, until the tops just begin to brown. Allow them to cool briefly before removing them from the pan. (To do so, loosen them with the tip of a knife if necessary.) Set aside.

For the chocolate coating, I suggest making two batches of coating so that it does not harden before you have used it all. Place half the chocolate bars in a microwave-safe bowl and cook on HIGH for 1 to 2 minutes, until melted. Stir in half the of vanilla. Stir until creamy.

Dip the cookies into the chocolate and place them on waxed paper to cool.

Crackerdoodles

brown rice flour

MAKES ABOUT 60 ONE-INCH SQUARE COOKIES

These cookies are a cross between a cracker and a snickerdoodle. When you need just a little something sweet, these cookies are perfect. My friends Erin and Michael Good are responsible for the creative title for these treats.

1/2 cup butter

1 1/2 cups brown rice flour, 185 grams

1/3 cup sugar, 75 grams

1/2 teaspoon baking soda

1/2 teaspoon salt

1 1/2 teaspoons xanthan gum

1 teaspoon vanilla extract

1/2 cup plain low-fat yogurt, 120 grams

TOPPING:

1 tablespoon sugar

1/2 teaspoon ground cinnamon

Preheat the oven to 375°F. Lightly grease a baking sheet.

In a medium-size bowl, combine all the batter ingredients, except the yogurt. Beat until fine crumbs form. Add the yogurt and beat until the dough comes together.

Press the dough as thinly and evenly as possible onto a baking sheet. Ideally, the dough will just about cover a 12 by 17-inch sheet pan, at 1/8-inch thickness or less. Use a sharp knife or pizza wheel to deeply score a grid pattern across the dough to create 1-inch squares. Use a fork to pierce holes throughout the tops of the cookies.

Combine the sugar and cinnamon. Sprinkle the dough with the cinnamon-sugar mixture.

Bake the cookies for 15 to 20 minutes, until the tops are golden brown. The cookies should be crisp. Break the cookies along the scored lines. Let cool on wire racks before serving.

Note: An empty salt shaker is ideal for mixing and sprinkling the cinnamon-sugar mixture.

| Egg-Free Cookies

Egg-Free Applesauce Bars

brown rice flour

MAKES 15 COOKIES

I designed these lower-fat, not-too-sweet bars to be reminiscent of bread pudding, but with a dense, cakelike texture. I hope you enjoy them as much as I enjoyed creating them! I've also included an optional cream cheese icing, should you like to counteract any low-fat benefits.

¹/₄ cup oil, 50 grams

1¹/₂ cups brown rice flour, 185 grams

¹/₃ cup honey, 105 grams

³/₄ cup applesauce

¹/₄ teaspoon baking soda

1 teaspoon baking powder

¹/₂ teaspoon salt

1 teaspoon vanilla extract

1 teaspoon ground nutmeg

³/₄ teaspoon xanthan gum

¹/₂ cup chopped raisins, 80 grams

ICING:

2 tablespoons shortening, 25 grams

¹/₂ cup confectioners' sugar, 60 grams

3 ounces cream cheese, 85 grams

Preheat the oven to 325°F. Lightly grease an 8-inch square baking pan.

In a medium-size bowl, combine the oil and brown rice flour. Beat well. Scrape down the sides of the mixing bowl at least once during mixing. Add the remaining cookie ingredients and mix well. The dough will be the consistency of thick batter.

Spread the dough evenly in the prepared pan. Bake for about 25 minutes until a toothpick tests cleanly. Cool.

For the icing, mix the ingredients together until well blended and spread it over the cookies. Let cool completely and cut into bars.

Egg-Free Banana Bars with Browned Butter Icing

brown rice flour

MAKES 15 COOKIES

The browned butter icing adds a nice contrast to this not-too-sweet cookie bar.

¹/₄ cup oil, 50 grams

1¹/₂ cups brown rice flour,
   185 grams

¹/₃ cup honey, 105 grams

³/₄ cup smashed bananas
   (2 to 3), or 6-ounce jar
   baby food bananas

¹/₄ teaspoon baking soda

1 teaspoon baking powder

¹/₂ teaspoon salt

1 teaspoon vanilla

³/₄ teaspoon xanthan gum

¹/₂ cup chopped nuts (optional)

FOR ICING:

¹/₄ cup butter

1¹/₂ tablespoons milk

1¹/₂ cups powdered sugar

Preheat the oven to 325°F. Lightly grease an 8-inch square pan.

In medium-size bowl, combine the oil and brown rice flour. Beat well to fully coat flour. Scrape down the sides of the mixing bowl at least once during mixing. Add the remaining ingredients and mix well. The dough will be the consistency of thick batter.

Spread in the prepared pan. Bake for approximately 25 minutes until a toothpick tests dry. Cool.

For icing, cook the butter over medium heat in a small pan, until lightly browned. The butter will become fragrant and almost nutty. Place the melted butter and the milk in the mixing bowl and gradually add the powdered sugar, while mixing, to form a smooth icing. Spread over the cookies.

Egg-Free Brownies

brown rice flour

MAKES ABOUT 15 BROWNIES

*These are moist, cakelike brownies, identical to egg-containing brownies . . .
no. Very tasty . . . yes!*

¹/₃ cup shortening, 70 grams

1¹/₂ cups brown rice flour,
185 grams

¹/₂ cup honey, 160 grams

¹/₄ cup sugar, 50 grams

¹/₃ cup unsweetened cocoa
powder, 30 grams

¹/₃ cup water, 65 grams

¹/₂ teaspoon baking soda

2 teaspoons baking powder

¹/₂ teaspoon salt

1 teaspoon vanilla extract

1 teaspoon xanthan gum

Preheat the oven to 325°F. Lightly grease an 8-inch square pan.

In a medium-size bowl, combine the shortening and brown rice flour. Beat well. Scrape down the sides of the mixing bowl at least once during mixing. Add the remaining ingredients and mix well. The brownie dough will be quite heavy in texture, but will come together with continued beating.

Spread the batter evenly in the prepared pan. Bake for about 25 minutes, until a toothpick tests cleanly. (The toothpick is unlikely to hold any batter, but will seem wet, when tested, if the brownies are not done.) When fully baked, the brownies will also begin to pull away from the sides of the pan.

Let cool completely and cut into bars.

Egg-Free Chocolate Chip Cookies

brown rice flour

MAKES ABOUT 30 COOKIES

For greater "brown sugar" flavor, you may wish to use a tablespoon of molasses
in place of 1 tablespoon of honey, use a darker color honey,
or simply enjoy as they are.

- 1/3 cup shortening, 70 grams
- 1³/₄ cups brown rice flour, 220 grams
- 1/2 cup honey, 160 grams
- 1/2 teaspoon baking soda
- 2 teaspoons baking powder
- 1/2 teaspoon salt
- 2 teaspoons vanilla extract
- 1 teaspoon pumpkin pie spice
- 1¹/₄ teaspoons xanthan gum
- 1/2 cup chocolate chips, 80 grams

Preheat the oven to 325°F. Lightly grease a cookie sheet.

In a medium-size bowl, combine the shortening and brown rice flour. Beat well. Scrape down the sides of the mixing bowl at least once during mixing. Add the remaining ingredients and mix well. The cookie dough will be quite heavy in texture.

Drop rounded teaspoonfuls of the dough onto the prepared pan. Using your fingertips, press them to 1/4-inch thickness. Bake the cookies for 7 to 9 minutes, until the bottom edges begin to brown and the tops take on a little color.

Egg-Free Chocolate Cookies

brown rice flour

MAKES ABOUT 30 COOKIES

These cookies are probably my favorite egg-free cookie in this book, although the chocolate chip cookies are a close second. This cookie has a very chewy brownie texture. For a more traditional texture, use honey instead of corn syrup and omit ¼ cup of the sugar.

¹/₃ cup shortening, 70 grams

1 ¹/₂ cups brown rice flour, 185 grams

¹/₂ cup corn syrup, 160 grams

¹/₂ cup sugar, 100 grams

¹/₃ cup unsweetened cocoa powder, 30 grams

¹/₂ teaspoon baking soda

1 teaspoon baking powder

¹/₂ teaspoon salt

1 teaspoon vanilla extract

³/₄ teaspoon xanthan gum

Preheat the oven to 325°F. Lightly grease a cookie sheet.

In a medium-size bowl, combine the shortening and brown rice flour. Beat well. Scrape down the sides of the mixing bowl at least once during mixing. Add the remaining ingredients and mix well. The cookie dough will be quite heavy in texture.

Drop rounded teaspoonfuls of the dough well apart onto the prepared pan. The cookies will spread during baking. Bake for 7 to 9 minutes until the bottom edges begin to brown and the tops take on a little color. Allow the cookies to cool briefly on the pan for easier removal.

Egg-Free Gingerbread Men

brown rice flour

MAKES ABOUT 30 COOKIES

This is a mild gingerbread cookie. For a richer flavor, substitute a few tablespoons of unsulfured molasses for a few tablespoons of the honey. Refrigeration of this dough is critical for rolling. For faster cookies, simply drop teaspoonsful of dough on the cookie sheet and bake.

1/3 cup shortening, 70 grams

1 3/4 cups brown rice flour, 220 grams

1/2 cup honey, 160 grams

1/4 teaspoon baking soda

1 teaspoon baking powder

1/2 teaspoon salt

1/2 teaspoon vanilla extract

1 1/4 teaspoons ground ginger

2 teaspoons xanthan gum

TOPPING:
Icing, decorative candies, and/or raisins

Preheat the oven to 350°F. Lightly grease a cookie sheet.

In a medium-size bowl, combine the shortening and brown rice flour. Beat well. Scrape down the sides of the mixing bowl at least once during mixing. Add the remaining ingredients and mix well. Once the dough comes together, continue beating for an additional minute or so to make the dough easier to handle. The dough will be very soft and ideally should be refrigerated for 30 minutes if you plan to roll it out and cut it, rather than make drop cookies. (The most adept at rolling cookies will prove me wrong on this point.)

Roll out the dough to a scant 1/4-inch thickness and cut it with gingerbread men cookie cutters. Place decorative candies or raisins on the cookies if desired. Bake for 7 to 9 minutes, until the edges just begin to brown. Let cool on wire racks. The cookies will stiffen while cooling. Decorate with icing, if desired.

Egg-Free Oatmeal Cookies

oats and brown rice flour
MAKES ABOUT 30 COOKIES

*These cookies are not-too-sweet, soft, and slightly chewy. They are the perfect
balance between light and heavy, being right in the middle.
I can't imagine not enjoying these.*

³/₄ cup rolled oats, 70 grams

¹/₃ cup shortening, 70 grams

1¹/₂ cups brown rice flour,
185 grams

¹/₂ cup honey, 160 grams

¹/₂ teaspoon baking soda

1 teaspoon baking powder

¹/₂ teaspoon salt

2 teaspoons vanilla extract

1 teaspoon xanthan gum

Preheat the oven to 325°F. Lightly grease a
cookie sheet.

Place the oats in a blender and pulse until they
are partially broken down. Pieces of all sizes
should remain. Set aside. In a medium-size
bowl, combine the shortening and brown
rice flour. Beat well. Scrape down the sides
of the mixing bowl at least once during mixing. Add the remaining ingredients, including the oats, and mix well. The cookie dough
will be very heavy to the beaters, but soft to
the touch.

Drop rounded teaspoonfuls of the dough onto
the prepared pan. Using your fingertips, press
them to ¹/₄-inch thickness. The cookies will
not spread much during baking. Bake for
8 to 10 minutes, until the bottom edges
begin to brown. Let cool on wire racks before serving.

Egg-Free Peanut Butter Cookies

brown rice flour

MAKES ABOUT 35 COOKIES

You can add ½ cup of chocolate chips to these if you've got a chocolate and peanut butter craving. Or keep them plain for an especially good traditional cookie! The slight undertone of the honey works nicely with the overall peanut butter flavor.

⅓ cup shortening, 70 grams

½ cup peanut butter, 140 grams

1½ cups brown rice flour, 185 grams

½ cup honey, 160 grams

½ teaspoon baking soda

2 teaspoons baking powder

½ teaspoon salt

1 teaspoon vanilla extract

1 teaspoon xanthan gum

Preheat the oven to 325°F. Lightly grease a cookie sheet.

In a medium-size bowl, combine the shortening, peanut butter, and brown rice flour. Beat well. Scrape down the sides of the mixing bowl at least once during mixing. Add the remaining ingredients and mix well. The cookie dough will be tacky and soft.

Drop rounded teaspoonfuls of the dough onto the prepared pan. Using the tines of a fork dipped in brown rice flour (or sprayed lightly with nonstick spray), press them to ¼-inch thickness. Bake for 8 to 10 minutes, until the bottom edges begin to brown and the tops take on a little color. Let cool on wire racks before serving.

Egg-Free Pumpkin Bars

brown rice flour
MAKES ABOUT 15 COOKIES

I developed these bars just before the Thanksgiving holiday. I love pumpkin pie and put that flavor in these quick cookie bars. These bars have a slightly dense, cakelike texture and are bright in flavor. Although a little icing would be pretty, a liberal sprinkling of confectioners' sugar is more than sufficient. If you want a slightly chewier texture, increase the xanthan gum to 1 teaspoon.

1/3 cup shortening, 70 grams

1 1/2 cups brown rice flour, 185 grams

1/2 cup honey, 160 grams

1/4 cup brown sugar, 50 grams

1/2 cup pumpkin puree, 100 grams

1/2 teaspoon baking soda

1 teaspoon baking powder

1/2 teaspoon salt

1 teaspoon vanilla extract

1 teaspoon pumpkin pie spice

3/4 teaspoon xanthan gum

TOPPING:
1/2 cup confectioners' sugar

Preheat the oven to 325°F. Lightly grease an 8-inch square pan.

In a medium-size bowl, combine the shortening and brown rice flour. Beat well. Scrape down the sides of the mixing bowl at least once during mixing. Add the remaining ingredients and mix well. The dough will be extremely soft.

Spread the dough evenly in the prepared pan. Bake for about 30 minutes, until a toothpick tests cleanly. (If the bars are not done, the toothpick is unlikely to hold any batter, but will seem wet.) Let cool.

Sprinkle the bars liberally with confectioners' sugar before slicing. Let cool, then cut into bars.

Note: These cookies will crumble if cut when still hot. Allow to cool for prettier bars!

Egg-Free Rolled Sugar Cookies

brown rice flour
MAKES ABOUT 30 COOKIES

As with the plain sugar cookies, corn syrup is used here for the neutral flavor base. The corn syrup gives almost a bit of chew to the cookie. And although they are sweet, they are not sugary sweet.

$1/3$ cup shortening, 70 grams

$1^3/4$ cups brown rice flour, 220 grams

$1/2$ cup corn syrup, 160 grams

$1/4$ cup sugar, 50 grams

$1/4$ teaspoon baking soda

1 teaspoon baking powder

$1/2$ teaspoon salt

1 teaspoon vanilla extract

$1^1/2$ teaspoons xanthan gum

TOPPING:
Icing and/or sprinkles

Preheat the oven to 350°F. Lightly grease a cookie sheet.

In a medium-size bowl, combine the shortening and brown rice flour. Beat well. Scrape down the sides of the mixing bowl at least once during mixing. Add the remaining ingredients and mix well. The cookie dough will be quite heavy in texture. Once the dough comes together, continue beating for an additional minute or so to make it easier to handle. The dough will be very soft and may be refrigerated for easier handling.

Roll out the dough to a scant $1/4$-inch thickness and cut it with your favorite cookie cutters. Top with sprinkles, if desired. Bake the cookies for 7 to 9 minutes, until the edges just begin to brown. Let cool on wire racks. Decorate with icing, if desired.

Egg-Free Spice Cookies

brown rice flour

MAKES ABOUT 30 COOKIES

This lightly flavored spice cookie is soft and pleasant.
I prefer it with the raisins, but I do chop them for what I think is better flavor.
The cookies have a soft yet tight crumb.

⅓ cup shortening, 70 grams

1¾ cups brown rice flour,
   220 grams

½ cup honey, 160 grams

½ teaspoon baking soda

2 teaspoons baking powder

½ teaspoon salt

1 teaspoon vanilla extract

1 teaspoon pumpkin pie spice

1¼ teaspoons xanthan gum

⅓ cup roughly chopped raisins
   (optional), 55 grams

Preheat the oven to 325°F. Lightly grease a cookie sheet.

In a medium-size bowl, combine the shortening and brown rice flour. Beat well. Scrape down the sides of the mixing bowl at least once during mixing. Add the remaining ingredients and mix well. The cookie dough will be quite heavy in texture.

Drop rounded teaspoonfuls of the dough onto the prepared pan. Use your fingertips to press them to ¼-inch thickness. Bake for 7 to 9 minutes, until the bottom edges begin to brown and the tops take on a little color. Let cool on wire racks before serving.

Egg-Free Sugar Cookies

brown rice flour

MAKES ABOUT 30 COOKIES

These cookies are a little light and crispy. Corn syrup is not as sweet as honey, but provides the neutral base needed for a plain sugar cookie. You may use a very, very light honey instead, but you will need to omit the sugar if you go that route.

¹/₃ cup shortening, 70 grams

1³/₄ cups brown rice flour, 220 grams

¹/₂ cup corn syrup, 160 grams

¹/₄ cup sugar, 50 grams

¹/₂ teaspoon baking soda

1 tablespoon baking powder

¹/₂ teaspoon salt

1 teaspoon vanilla extract

1 teaspoon xanthan gum

TOPPING:
2 tablespoons sugar or sprinkles

Preheat the oven to 350°F. Lightly grease a cookie sheet.

In a medium-size bowl, combine the shortening and brown rice flour. Beat well. Scrape down the sides of the mixing bowl at least once during mixing. Add the remaining ingredients and mix well. The cookie dough will be quite heavy in texture.

Drop rounded teaspoonfuls of the dough onto the prepared pan. Press to ¹/₄-inch thickness with your fingertips. Sprinkle the tops with sugar or sprinkles, as desired. Bake the cookies for 7 to 9 minutes, until the bottom edges just begin to brown. Let cool on wire racks before serving.

Fruitcake Nuggets

cornstarch or potato starch

MAKES ABOUT 20 COOKIES

These cookies would be great to make at the same time as the Almond Joy–Style Cookies (page 144) as each use just ½ cup of sweetened condensed milk. These will be enjoyed by most guests at your holiday party, not just the fruitcake lover!

1 (7-ounce) bag sweetened flaked coconut (2²/₃ cups)

2 tablespoons cornstarch or potato starch

¹/₂ cup sweetened condensed milk

1 cup candied fruit

1 cup chopped walnuts

1 teaspoon vanilla extract

Preheat the oven to 325°F. Lightly grease a mini-muffin pan.

In a medium-size bowl, combine the coconut and starch. Stir well. Add the remaining ingredients and mix well. Drop rounded teaspoonfuls of the dough into the cups of the prepared pan. With moist fingertips, press down the cookie dough a little so that the cookies stick together.

Bake for 13 to 15 minutes, until the tops just begin to brown. Allow the cookies to cool briefly before removing them from the pan. You can loosen them with the tip of a knife if necessary.

Orange-Cream Cheese Tassies

brown rice flour

MAKES ABOUT 24 TASSIES

Soft, orange cheesecakey filling surrounded by a crisp sugar cookie cup.

$\frac{1}{3}$ cup shortening, 70 grams

1$\frac{3}{4}$ cups brown rice flour,
    220 grams

$\frac{1}{2}$ cup corn syrup, 160 grams

$\frac{1}{4}$ cup sugar, 50 grams

$\frac{1}{4}$ teaspoon baking soda

1 teaspoon baking powder

$\frac{1}{2}$ teaspoon salt

1 teaspoon vanilla extract

1$\frac{1}{2}$ teaspoons xanthan gum

FILLING:
1 (8-ounce) package cream cheese

$\frac{1}{2}$ cup confectioners' sugar,
    60 grams

$\frac{1}{3}$ cup orange marmalade,
    120 grams

Preheat the oven to 350°F. Lightly grease a 24-count mini-muffin pan.

For the tart shells, in a medium-size bowl, combine the shortening and brown rice flour. Beat well. Scrape down the sides of the mixing bowl at least once during mixing. Add the remaining dough ingredients and mix well. The cookie dough will be quite heavy in texture. Once the dough comes together, continue beating it for an additional minute or so to make the dough easier to handle; it will be very soft.

Drop rounded teaspoonfuls of the dough into the cups of the prepared pan and press the center with the back of a spoon to evenly form tart shells. Set aside.

For the filling, combine all the ingredients and mix very well. Place rounded teaspoonfuls of the filling into the center of the shells.

Bake the cookies for about 9 minutes, until the shell is golden and the filling is set. Allow the cookies to cool in the pan for about 5 minutes, for easier removal. Let cool on wire racks before serving.

| Egg-Free Cookies

Pepper Jack Cookies

brown rice flour

MAKES ABOUT 55 COOKIES

To the palate, these cookies begin as a delicate, slightly sweet cookie, followed by a bit of growing, mellow heat. The salt adds to the play on the tongue. These are great served with a glass of wine or as an unexpected treat on a cookie tray.

4 ounces pepper Jack cheese, finely grated

¹/₄ cup butter, chopped in small chunks

²/₃ cup brown rice flour, 85 grams

¹/₄ cup sugar, 50 grams

¹/₂ teaspoon xanthan gum

¹/₂ teaspoon baking powder

¹/₂ teaspoon salt

TOPPING:
Salt

Preheat the oven to 375°F. Lightly grease a cookie sheet.

In a medium-size bowl, combine all the ingredients. Beat (or mix with your fingertips) until the dough forms a soft ball.

Roll out the dough to ¹/₄-inch thickness. Cut it into cookies with a 1-inch cookie cutter and place them on the prepared pan. Bake for 8 to 10 minutes, until the bottoms of the cookies are tinged with color. Let cool on wire racks before serving.

Note: Be careful as you bake these cookies, as they are very easy to burn on the bottom. The browning will barely be visible from a side view.

9

Cookies Made with Other Gluten-Free Flours

In baking gluten-free, we are often tempted to purchase many different flours, either because they are new and exciting (as was the case when coconut flour first came out), for nutritional content (such as bean flours, or certain pseudograins), or simply because they are called for in a blend. It is hard to get to know the nature of a flour when it is just one of many. The old theory that you must use a blend to bake good foods hasn't helped, either.

While the other recipes in this book call for either brown rice flour or sorghum flour, the cookies in this chapter use a variety of flours, just one at a time, to let their character show through. We may even make a dent in that tower of flours you've accumulated over time. You can make a cookie out of almost any gluten-free flour. But that doesn't mean you want to eat them. And, for that reason, a number of stronger-tasting flours, such as soy and teff, have simply not been utilized in this chapter.

Please be sure to try the Chocolate Crinkles made with garbanzo bean flour. They are one of my favorites. Oatmeal, potato starch, cornstarch, and even tapioca starch do a cookie proud in this chapter!

And, finally, at the risk of being extremely blunt, I would describe the flavor of coconut flour on its own as tasting like tropical dirt. Used with other tropical flavors, it is much more palatable. It is also not very responsive to leavening. However, it does make a very pretty, flat cookie. It would be ideal to use in making cookie ornaments: expensive, but ideal.

If you have the time, I strongly encourage you to bake with just one flour at a time. It surely helps in figuring out what you like in a flour, what suits your tummy, and ultimately which flours are worth the price.

Blueberry-Cranberry Jumbles

potato starch

MAKES ABOUT 25 COOKIES

A bright and healthy change from chocolate chip, the fruit flavor in this cookie shines. If you are a fan of blueberry pancakes, try the recipe with just the dried blueberries. Tasty! The cookie base is very tender, quite sweet, and a good contrast to the chewy bits of fruit.

1/3 cup oil, 65 grams

1/2 cup sugar, 100 grams

1 cup potato starch, 155 grams

1 egg

1/4 teaspoon baking soda

1/2 teaspoon salt

1/2 teaspoon xanthan gum

1 teaspoon vanilla extract

1/3 cup coarsely chopped dried blueberries, 60 grams

1/3 cup coarsely chopped dried, sweetened cranberries, 40 grams

Preheat the oven to 350°F. Lightly grease a cookie sheet.

In a medium-size bowl, combine the oil and sugar. Beat well. Add the potato starch and beat well. Scrape down the sides of the mixing bowl at least once during mixing. Add the remaining ingredients, except the blueberries and cranberries, and mix well. The dough will be like a thick cake batter. Stir in the berries.

Drop rounded teaspoonfuls of the dough onto the prepared pan. Bake the cookies for 8 to 9 minutes, until the bottom edges are browned. Let cool on wire racks before serving.

Chocolate Biscotti

oat flour

MAKES ABOUT 30 COOKIES

A simple, traditional biscotti, adorned with just a little flavored icing. Nuts, chocolate chips, or other tasty bits would make a nice addition.

¹/₃ cup shortening, 70 grams

¹/₄ cup sugar, 100 grams

1 cup oat flour, 120 grams

¹/₃ cup unsweetened cocoa powder, 30 grams

2 eggs

¹/₄ teaspoon baking soda

1 teaspoon baking powder

¹/₂ teaspoon salt

¹/₂ teaspoon xanthan gum

1 teaspoon vanilla extract

Pinch of cayenne (optional)

TOPPING:

²/₃ cup confectioners' sugar

1 tablespoon of your favorite gluten-free liqueur (or water)

Preheat the oven to 350°F. Lightly grease a cookie sheet.

In a medium-size bowl, combine the shortening and sugar. Beat well. Add the remaining ingredients and mix well. Scrape down the sides of the mixing bowl at least once during mixing. The dough will be soft and heavy.

Divide the dough in half. Shape each portion into a flattened log about ½-inch tall and place on the prepared pan. (This is a good opportunity to mix in any nuts, chocolate chips, or other tasty goodies, if desired.) Do the same with the other half of the dough.

Bake the logs for 20 minutes. Let cool completely. Cut each log into slices about ½-inch thick and place these back on the prepared pan. Bake the biscotti for an additional 10 to 15 minutes, until quite dry. Let cool again.

Combine the confectioners' sugar and liqueur in a small cup and stir to dissolve. Spread the mixture over the tops of the cookies.

Chocolate Cookies, Dairy-Free

cornmeal

MAKES ABOUT 30 COOKIES

Corn teams up with chocolate for a crisp, tender cookie that is almost chewy, with a hint of grit. This is a chocolate cookie that will please most anyone. Add the optional drizzle of chocolate to make them prettier if you like.

1/3 cup shortening, 65 grams

3/4 cup sugar, 150 grams

1 1/4 cups cornmeal, 150 grams (120 grams per cup)

1/3 cup cocoa, 30 grams

2 eggs

1/4 teaspoon baking soda

2 teaspoons baking powder

1/2 teaspoon salt

1/2 teaspoon xanthan gum

1 teaspoon vanilla extract

TOPPING (OPTIONAL):
2 ounces chocolate

Preheat the oven to 350°F. Lightly grease a cookie sheet.

In a medium-size bowl, combine the shortening and sugar. Beat well. Add the cornmeal and beat well. Scrape down the sides of the mixing bowl at least once during mixing. Add the remaining ingredients and mix well. The dough will be gooey and pasty.

Drop rounded teaspoonfuls of the dough onto the prepared baking pan. Using wet fingertips, press to 1/4-inch thickness.

Bake for 8 to 10 minutes, until the edges look dry and the tops are slightly crackled. Do not overbake. Allow the cookies to cool on wire racks. Place the chocolate in a microwave-proof plastic cup and cook on HIGH for 1 minute, then drizzle the tops of the cookies with the melted chocolate, if desired.

Chocolate Crinkles

garbanzo bean flour
MAKES ABOUT 25 COOKIES

This cookie has a rich chocolate flavor and is a little chewy. You will be hard-pressed to identify the bean flour. All in all, a very good cookie.

1/3 cup oil, 65 grams

1/2 cup sugar, 100 grams

1 1/4 cups garbanzo bean flour, 135 grams

1/3 cup unsweetened cocoa powder, 30 grams

1 egg

1/4 teaspoon baking soda

1/2 teaspoon salt

1/2 teaspoon xanthan gum

1 teaspoon vanilla extract

2 tablespoons water

TOPPING:
1/4 cup confectioners' sugar

Preheat the oven to 350°F. Lightly grease a cookie sheet.

In a medium-size bowl, combine the oil and sugar. Beat well. Add the garbanzo bean flour and cocoa and beat well. Scrape down the sides of the mixing bowl at least once during mixing. Add the remaining ingredients and mix well. The dough will be heavy and sticky.

Place the confectioners' sugar in small bowl. Drop rounded teaspoonfuls of the dough into the confectioners' sugar and roll to coat well. Place them onto the prepared pan and use your fingertips to press them to about 1/4-inch thickness.

Bake for 8 to 9 minutes, until the tops are dry. The cookies spread little, if any, during baking. Let cool on wire racks before serving.

Cloud Cookies

cornstarch
MAKES ABOUT 25 COOKIES

Pillow soft and not too sweet. These cookies are topped with finely chopped chocolate or nuts. They are both plain and sophisticated at the same time.

$^1/_3$ cup oil, 65 grams

$^1/_3$ cup sugar, 75 grams

$1^1/_4$ cups cornstarch, 155 grams

1 egg yolk

2 egg whites

$^1/_4$ teaspoon baking soda

$^1/_2$ teaspoon salt

$^1/_2$ teaspoon xanthan gum

$^1/_2$ teaspoon vanilla extract

TOPPING:
$^1/_2$ cup finely chopped chocolate chips

and/or

$^1/_2$ cup finely chopped nuts

Preheat the oven to 350°F. Lightly grease a cookie sheet.

In a medium-size bowl, combine the oil and sugar. Beat well. Add the cornstarch and beat well. Scrape down the sides of the mixing bowl at least once during mixing. Add the remaining ingredients and mix well. The dough will be as thin as cake batter.

Drop rounded teaspoonfuls of the dough well apart onto the prepared pan. Sprinkle the tops with chocolate bits and/or nuts. Bake for 8 to 9 minutes, until the bottom edges are browned. The cookies will spread during baking. Let cool on wire racks before serving.

Note: I like to melt a small chocolate bar and spread it on the top of the cookies and sprinkle them with nuts.

Coconut Chip Cookies

coconut flour
MAKES ABOUT 30 COOKIES

The chopped coconut and chocolate chips make this cookie come together. Without those embellishments, these cookies would have a "muddy" coconut undertone that doesn't shine as well. (But alone, that base cookie would make a good substitute for the base cookies in the great fake Samoas, page 102).

1/3 cup oil, 65 grams

1/2 cup sugar, 100 grams

1 cup coconut flour, 140 grams

2 eggs

1/4 teaspoon baking soda

1 teaspoon baking powder

1/2 teaspoon salt

1/2 teaspoon xanthan gum

1 teaspoon vanilla extract

1/4 cup water

3/4 cup coarsely chopped chocolate chips

1/2 cup coarsely chopped sweetened flaked coconut

Preheat the oven to 350°F. Lightly grease a cookie sheet.

In a medium-size bowl, combine all the ingredients and mix well. Scrape down the sides of the mixing bowl at least once during mixing. The dough will come together and be very thick and soft.

Roll out to 1/4-inch thickness and cut into desired shapes. Bake for 8 to 9 minutes, until lightly browned at the edges. Let cool on wire racks before serving.

Fortune Cookies and Pirouettes

tapioca starch

MAKES ABOUT 15 COOKIES

In making these, the goal is to have a pliable disk of cookie that can be quickly shaped before it cools into a crisp cookie. Please know that these cookies will be an effort in patience and diligence to get them baked for just the right amount of time—too long and the cookie will be burnt; too short and the cookie will have an unwanted softness to the bite. Baking several single test cookies should give you the exact timing for your oven. Remember to include great fortunes!

2 egg whites

1/2 cup sugar, 100 grams

1 cup tapioca starch, 90 grams

1 tablespoon shortening

3 tablespoons milk

1/4 teaspoon xanthan gum

Pinch of baking soda

Preheat the oven to 325°F. Lightly grease a cookie sheet. Prepare slips of paper with fortunes, if desired.

Mix all the ingredients in a medium-size bowl, until well blended. (A whisk is useful for this.) Be sure no lumps remain.

For each cookie, drop scant tablespoonfuls of the batter well apart onto the prepared pan. The batter will be thin. If the batter thickens upon standing, spread it out into a 3-inch circle. Place up to four rounds of batter on the prepared pan.

Bake for 8 to 10 minutes, until the edges of the cookies are golden brown. The bottom of the cookies will also be browned.

(continues on next page)

| Cookies Made with Other Gluten-Free Flours

For fortune cookies: Remove a cookie from the pan with a spatula and place a fortune in the center. Fold the cookie in half and then bring the two ends together (while pushing the center fold area with your finger) to shape the cookie. Allow to cool.

For pirouette cookies: Remove a cookie from the pan with a spatula and quickly roll the cookie around a pencil or similar thin item. Let cool on wire racks before serving.

Note: Tapioca starch measures quite differently from the amounts listed on the package. If at all possible, please measure your flour by weight.

Iced Oatmeal Cookies

oats and oat flour

MAKES ABOUT 30 COOKIES

This cookie is fashioned after the Iced Oatmeal Cookies from Trader Joe's. They are hard, crispy, and full of both vanilla and cinnamon flavors. Please remember to use only safe oats in your gluten-free baking!

1 cup rolled oats, 85 grams

1/3 cup shortening, 70 grams

1/2 cup sugar, 100 grams

1 cup oat flour, 120 grams

1 egg

1/4 teaspoon baking soda

1/2 teaspoon salt

1/2 teaspoon xanthan gum

1 teaspoon vanilla extract

1/2 teaspoon ground cinnamon

TOPPING:

2/3 cup confectioners' sugar

1 tablespoon water

Preheat the oven to 350°F. Lightly grease a cookie sheet.

Place the oats in a blender and pulse until most pieces are about a quarter of the original size. In a medium-size bowl, combine the shortening and sugar. Beat well. Add the cut oats and the remaining ingredients and mix well. Scrape down the sides of the mixing bowl at least once during mixing. The dough will be soft and heavy.

Drop rounded teaspoonfuls of the dough onto the prepared pan. Press them with your fingertips (or the base of a glass) to about 1/8-inch thickness.

Bake the cookies for 10 to 11 minutes, until lightly browned. Let cool on wire racks.

Combine the confectioners' sugar and water in a small cup. Stir to dissolve. Spread the mixture over the tops of the cookies.

Love Letter Rolled Chocolate Sugar Cookies

tapioca starch

MAKES ABOUT 14 COOKIES

Cut into mini envelopes, these cookies are a pretty way to enjoy a crisp, tender, chocolaty cookie. Decorate with a little icing to bring the envelopes to life.

$1/_3$ cup shortening, 70 grams

$1/_2$ cup sugar, 100 grams

$1 1/_2$ cups tapioca starch, 135 grams

$1/_3$ cup unsweetened cocoa powder, 30 grams

1 egg plus 1 egg yolk

$1/_4$ teaspoon baking soda

$1/_2$ teaspoon salt

$1/_2$ teaspoon xanthan gum

1 teaspoon vanilla extract

Preheat the oven to 350°F. Lightly grease a cookie sheet.

In medium-size bowl, combine the shortening and sugar. Beat well. Add the tapioca starch and beat well. Scrape down the sides of the mixing bowl at least once during mixing. Add the remaining ingredients and mix well. The dough will just come together and be quite heavy.

Roll out the dough to ⅛-inch thickness and cut into 2 by 4-inch rectangles. Bake for 8 to 9 minutes, until the edges take on a little color and the tops are dry. Let cool on wire racks. Decorate with icing to mimic a letter or envelope.

Oatmeal Cookies

cornstarch and oats

MAKES ABOUT 30 COOKIES

These cookies are soft with simple vanilla flavoring. Feel free to spice them up with a little cinnamon and/or nutmeg! Or, add my kids' favorite: chocolate chips.

⅓ cup oil, 65 grams

½ cup brown sugar, 100 grams

1 ¼ cups cornstarch, 155 grams

⅔ cup rolled oats

2 eggs

½ teaspoon baking soda

½ teaspoon salt

½ teaspoon xanthan gum

½ teaspoon vanilla extract

1 cup chocolate chips (optional)

Preheat the oven to 350°F. Lightly grease a cookie sheet.

In a medium-size bowl, combine the oil and sugar. Beat well. Add the cornstarch and beat well. Scrape down the sides of the mixing bowl at least once during mixing. Add the remaining ingredients and mix well. The dough will seem like a thick, sticky batter.

Drop rounded teaspoonfuls of the dough well apart onto the prepared pan. With moistened fingertips, press them to ¼-inch thickness. Bake for 8 to 9 minutes, until the bottom edges are browned. The cookies will spread during baking. Let cool on wire racks before serving.

Pumpkin Cookies

garbanzo bean flour
MAKES ABOUT 25 COOKIES

This cookie is a moist, light, and nicely spiced cookie. But this is not raw dough that you will want to nibble on. Not even a little bit—it's beany! Bean flour is a taste that's not for everyone. However, baked and cooled, this is a pretty good cookie.

1/3 cup oil, 65 grams

1/2 cup sugar, 100 grams

1 1/4 cups garbanzo bean flour, 135 grams

1 egg

1/2 cup pumpkin puree

1/4 teaspoon baking soda

1 teaspoon baking powder

1/2 teaspoon salt

1/2 teaspoon xanthan gum

1 teaspoon vanilla extract

1 1/2 teaspoons pumpkin pie spice

1/2 cup coarsely chopped raisins

Preheat the oven to 350°F. Lightly grease a cookie sheet.

In a medium-size bowl, combine the oil and sugar. Beat well. Add the garbanzo bean flour and beat well. Scrape down the sides of the mixing bowl at least once during mixing. Add the remaining ingredients and mix well. The dough will be soft and not too heavy.

Drop rounded teaspoonfuls of the dough onto the prepared pan. Press them with your fingertips to a scant 1/4-inch thickness.

Bake the cookies for 8 to 9 minutes, until the edges are lightly browned. Let cool on wire racks before serving.

Rolled Sugar Cookies, Dairy-Free

cornmeal

MAKES ABOUT 30 COOKIES

This gritty flour makes a very tasty cookie. Not surprisingly, the cookie tastes pleasantly of corn. Sprinkles are nice, but the addition of a light icing substantially diminishes the corn flavor.

1/3 cup shortening, 65 grams

1/2 cup sugar, 100 grams

1 1/2 cups cornmeal, 180 grams (120 grams per cup)

1 egg

1/4 teaspoon baking soda

1 teaspoon baking powder

1/2 teaspoon salt

1 teaspoon xanthan gum

1 teaspoon vanilla extract

TOPPING (OPTIONAL): Sprinkles or colored sugar

Preheat the oven to 350°F. Lightly grease a cookie sheet.

In a medium-size bowl, combine the shortening and sugar. Beat well. Add the cornmeal and beat well. Scrape down the sides of the mixing bowl at least once during mixing. Add the remaining ingredients and mix well. Continue beating until the dough comes together.

Roll out the dough to 1/8-inch thickness (for crispier cookies) or to 1/4-inch thickness (for a bit softer) and cut it with a 2-inch round cookie cutter (or other cookie cutter of your choice).

Place the cookies on the prepared cookie sheet and top with sprinkles or colored sugar, if desired. Bake for 8 to 10 minutes, until they have the slightest hint of color.

Let cool on wire racks.

Rosettes

potato starch and cornstarch
MAKES ABOUT 100 COOKIES

There are times when some flours are just better suited to do a job. This is especially true when a light batter is fried. Enjoy these pretty, light cookies with just a bit of confectioners' sugar sprinkled on top. Rosettes are the "cookie" version of a funnel cake. In making these, I used an antique rosette mold from my mother-in-law, Lucile.

½ cup potato starch, 80 grams

½ cup cornstarch, 65 grams

1 tablespoon sugar

¼ teaspoon baking soda

1 teaspoon baking powder

½ teaspoon xanthan gum

½ teaspoon vanilla extract

Pinch of salt

1 egg

⅔ cup milk

FOR FRYING:
2 cups canola oil

TOPPING:
½ cup confectioners' sugar

Prior to frying, heat the oil to 370°F.

In a medium bowl, combine the potato starch, cornstarch, sugar, baking soda, baking powder, xanthan gum, vanilla, and salt. Add the egg. Slowly add the milk, mixing well to remove all lumps. Transfer the batter to a shallow bowl. The batter will thicken a lot over the course of making the rosettes; this is fine.

Dip the rosette iron into hot oil to heat for about 30 seconds. (Lift to drain off excess oil.) Then, dip the rosette iron into the batter to coat it most of the way up its sides. (It is very likely that you will need to dip, lift up, and dip again to get sufficient coating.) Do not cover the top of the iron or the cookie will not slide off. Return the iron to the hot oil and fry the rosette for 25 to 30 seconds, until golden brown. Lift it from the oil and, using a fork, gently ease the rosette from the iron and place it on paper towels to drain. Continue until all the batter is used.

Dust the tops with confectioners' sugar.

| Cookies Made with Other Gluten-Free Flours

Spritz

potato starch

MAKES ABOUT 36 COOKIES

Pretty, delicate, and delicious.
Dip them in dark chocolate for a special treat!

¹/₃ cup shortening, 70 grams

¹/₃ cup sugar, 75 grams

1 cup potato starch, 155 grams

1 egg

¹/₄ teaspoon baking soda

¹/₂ teaspoon salt

³/₄ teaspoon xanthan gum

1 teaspoon vanilla extract

Preheat the oven to 350°F. Lightly grease a cookie sheet.

In a medium-size bowl, combine the shortening and sugar. Beat well. Add the potato starch and beat well. Scrape down the sides of the mixing bowl at least once during mixing. Add the remaining ingredients and mix well. The dough will be soft.

Using a pastry bag, pipe the cookies well apart onto the prepared pan. As the cookies spread a lot during baking, be sure to leave room between the cookies. Bake for 8 to 9 minutes, until the bottom edges are browned. Let cool on wire racks before serving.

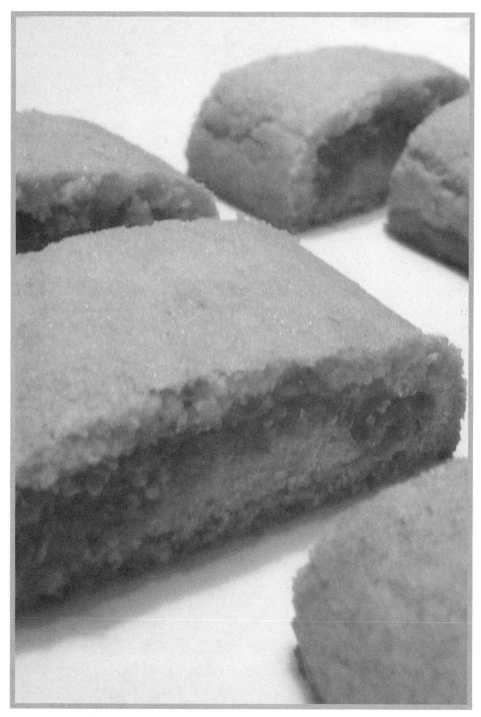

Fig Newton–Style Cookies, page 97

Appendix

Gluten-Free Resources

National Gluten-Free Support Groups

American Celiac Society

www.americanceliacsociety.org
PO Box 23455
New Orleans, LA 70183
504-737-3293

Celiac Disease Foundation

www.celiac.org
13251 Ventura Boulevard, #1
Studio City, CA 91604
818-990-2354

Celiac Sprue Association/USA Inc.

www.csaceliacs.org
PO Box 31700
Omaha, NE 68131
877-CSA-4CSA

The Gluten Intolerance Group of North America

www.gluten.net
31214 124th Ave SE
Seattle, WA 98092
253-833-6655

Local Celiac Support Groups

Celiac.com

www.celiac.com
Scroll down the home page to locate index, then click on support groups.

Gluten-Free Mail Order Suppliers

We are fortunate that there are now numerous gluten-free food suppliers in the United States. Even better, most of what you need can be found at your local grocery store or health food store. A Web search of "gluten-free foods" will

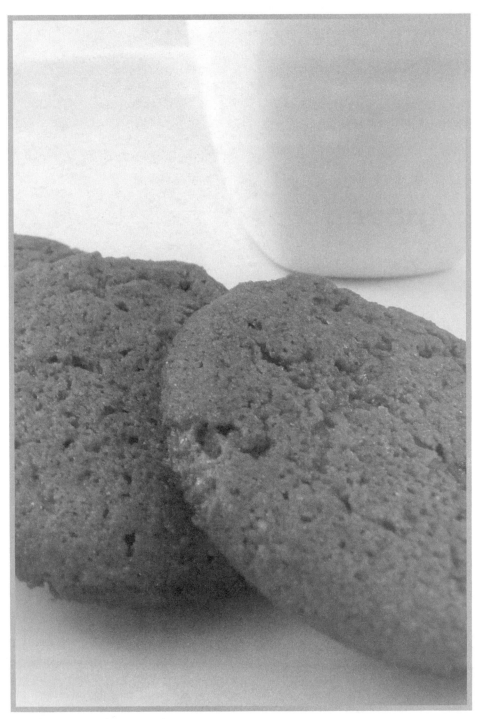

Hot Chocolate Cookies, page 30

Gluten-Free Mail Order
Suppliers *(continued)*

give you hundreds of options for high-quality gluten-free food suppliers, but you really only need a few. Here are several of the best:

Amazon.com

www.amazon.com

A surprising home to many gluten-free foods and baking supplies. You'll save if ordering in quantity, but be sure you like the item before you order in bulk. Many gluten-free books can be ordered quite reasonably there as well.

Breads from Anna by Gluten Evolution, LLC

www.glutenevolution.com
Iowa City, Iowa
319-354-3886
877-354-3886

This small company has mixes for some very good breads. In my opinion, they made the best overall bread at the last conference I attended. And, that is why they are listed here.

Celiac.com

www.celiac.com

Home to the "celiac mall," which includes numerous suppliers of gluten-free foods, books, and so on.

The Gluten-Free Pantry

www.glutenfree.com
PO Box 840
Glastonbury, CT 06033
860-633-3826

Gluten-free baking supplies and mixes.

Ener-G Foods

www.energyfoods.com
PO Box 84487
5960 1st Avenue South
Seattle, WA 98124
800-331-5222

Manufacturers of Safe Oats

Bob's Red Mill

www.bobsredmill.com
5209 S.E. International Way
Milwaukie, OR 97222
800-553-2258

Gluten-free oats, baking supplies, etc.

Gifts of Nature, Inc.

www.giftsofnature.net
810 7th St. E, #17
Polson, MT 59860
888-275-0003

Cream Hill Estates

www.creamhillestates.com
9633 rue Clement
LaSalle, Quebec
Canada H8R 4B4
514-363-2066
1-866-727-3628

Gluten Free Oats

www.glutenfreeoats.com
578 Lane 9
Powell, WY 82435
307-754-2058

My Favorite Gluten-Free Books

Celiac Disease: A Hidden Epidemic by Dr. Peter Green. Dr. Green takes the reader through the sometimes complicated and intimidating world of gluten-free living. The serious medical content of this book is softened by Dr. Green's straightforward, down-to-earth writing style. The questions and struggles of real patients peppered throughout the work put a human face on the disease.

The Gluten-Free Kitchen by Roben Ryberg. I am naturally biased toward my first book. Several of my very favorite recipes reside there, including angel and chiffon cakes, breakfast gravies, raised doughnuts, and a number of main courses.

You Won't Believe It's Gluten-Free!: 500 Delicious, Foolproof Recipes for Healthy Living by Roben Ryberg. I am most proud of this work because it meets so many dietary needs by using just one flour at a time. From appetizers through desserts, just one gluten-free flour can be amazing!

My Favorite Gluten-Free Magazine

Living Without

> www.livingwithout.com
> PO Box 2126
> Northbrook, IL 60065

Additional Resources for the Gluten-Free Community

In addition to the national and local support groups, www.celiac.com is a wonderful resource for medical studies, recipes, diagnosis steps, and so on.

My favorite online discussion board is www.forums.delphi.com/celiac/start. Most important, they have adopted a "zero-tolerance" policy for inclusion of any gluten in the diet (i.e., simply picking croutons off a salad is not safe!). It is a great place to talk with other individuals who live the celiac diet every day. There is no fee for basic membership. You will sometimes find me there.

Another very good on-line discussion board is www.glutenfreeforum.com.

For vacation getaways without worry, visit www.bobandruths.com.

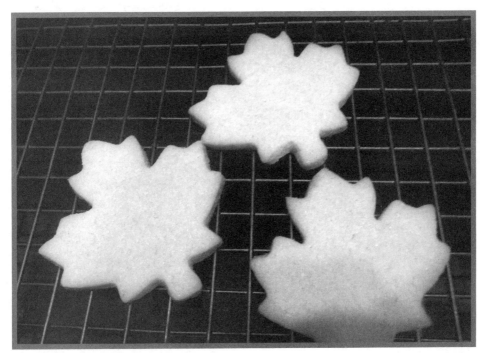

Maple Leaf Cookies, page 113

Note: Thousands of helpful organizations, companies and Web sites are available to the gluten-free community. Mountains of information are readily available. After making your home safe, the next step should be joining a support group—whether national, local, or online—and learning more. And, if you're not the support-group type, learn more by visiting the Web sites included in this appendix.

Index

A

B

H

I

J

L

M

| Index

S